Harmony in
Healing

Harmony in Healing

The Theoretical Basis of Ancient and Medieval Medicine

James J. Garber

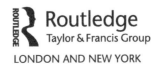

Routledge
Taylor & Francis Group

LONDON AND NEW YORK

First published 2008 by Transaction Publishers

2 Park Square, Milton Park, Abingdon, Oxfordshire OX14 4RN
711 Third Avenue, New York, NY 10017

Routledge is an imprint of the Taylor & Francis Group, an informa business

First issued in paperback 2017

Library of Congress Catalog Number: 2007052484

Library of Congress Cataloging-in-Publication Data

Garber, James J.
    Harmony in healing : the theoretical basis of ancient and medieval medi-
cine / James J. Garber.
       p. ; cm.
    Includes bibliographical references and index.
    ISBN 978-1-4128-0692-3 (alk. paper)
       1. Medicine, Ancient. 2. Medicine, Medieval. 3. Medicine--Philoso-
phy--History. I. Title.
    [DNLM: 1. History, Ancient. 2. History, Medieval. 3. Philosophy, Medi-
cal--history. WZ 51 G213h 2008]

R135.G37 2008
610.1--dc22

                                                              2007052484

ISBN 13: 978-1-4128-0692-3 (hbk)
ISBN 13: 978-1-138-51053-1 (pbk)

Dedicated to my wife Rachel and our adult family:
Ann, Clare, Jim, Suzanne, Dave, John and Pete

Contents

Preface

Several years ago I was faced with the need to find a topic for my master's thesis in astronomy and it became apparent that there was an historical and philosophical connection between medicine and the stars. I have spent most of my professional life in medicine. However, I had also maintained a continual interest in astronomy along with philosophy and history. I thought rather than a technical astronomical thesis, an "armchair" topic might be more to my liking at this stage of life I had already spent many (frigid) hours peering through a telescope and working through complex mathematical problems. It was time to relax a bit. For a history of astronomy course I had researched the topic of Cepheid variables and found this comer of astronomy filled with all kinds of philosophical and religious overtones. It was soon evident that medicine, too, was intricately entangled with astronomy. Finally, it seemed possible for me to mix into one scholarly "stew" all those interests that had been simmering in my consciousness for so many years.

From the master's thesis grew a doctoral dissertation and now this book. I hope it will shed light on both astronomy and medicine as well as provide a better understanding of history and human nature.

James J. Garber

Acknowledgements

I want to thank the many teachers I've had over the years—too many to list—but all very important in the academics that led up to the creation of this book. It has been a long, enjoyable journey. Special thanks must go to my doctoral advisor, Professor Naomi Lichtenberg, who not only gave me direction but also helped develop the writing skills necessary for such a work. Thanks also to Professors John R. Christianson and Marie Maher who reviewed the dissertation. The Rochester, Minnesota Public Library was instrumental in obtaining needed resources in a timely manner. And to my wife and best friend I owe thanks for her encouragement, suggestions and the many hours she spent editing all my writings over the past six years.

To my breakfast friends, all college teachers, I am grateful for their continuing stimulation and support. Special thanks to Marie Miller with her sharp eyes and keen mind was invaluable in making this book presentable. Lastly, appreciation goes to Laurence Mintz of Transaction Publishing for his patience in this my first literary foray.

I also wish to express my gratitude for the most gracious permission of Her Majesty, Queen Elizabeth II, for the use of the reproduction of the Leonardo da Vinci drawing (Fig. 6.1) from the Windsor Castle Library.

Introduction

Medicine and astronomy appear at first glance to be the original "odd couple." However, as we shall see, it was a union whose progeny were to populate the Western world for more than two millennia. They are, arguably, the oldest of all the sciences,[1] which may, in part, explain this odd pairing. From an historical perspective, their marriage and mutual influences are undeniable.[2] Cosmology and cosmogony, as "natural philosophical" aspects of astronomy, have gone hand in hand with the science of medicine from time immemorial. Indeed, medicine and the pseudoscience of astrology were for centuries inseparable. The ancients began the embryonic search for answers to questions that had puzzled humans for unknown eons. No systematic approach to the nature of the Universe was undertaken until the Sumerians, Babylonians and, later, the Greeks began the quest for "wisdom"—to use Aristotle's term.[3] The Greeks, beginning with Thales in the sixth century B.C.E., sought a unifying principle to explain the world as a whole. Because cosmology and medicine were among the few known sciences at the time, it was natural that these two apparently disparate disciplines should be combined to provide the theoretical foundations of medicine—foundations that were to survive for nearly 2,400 years. This scientific structure rested firmly on the ancient principles of cosmology, astronomy, and the concept of universal harmony. This book tells the tale of these theoretical underpinnings and how they influenced humankind's efforts to maintain health and fight disease. It was a futile effort because the system was fundamentally flawed. Nonetheless, it lingered for centuries beyond what common sense tells us it should have.

No comprehensive analysis of the cosmology-medicine relationship has been undertaken in the astronomical or medical literature. For better or (mostly) for worse, these cosmological principles have had profound effects on the theory and practice of medicine over the centuries. It is time for historians, astronomers, physicians, and philosophers to acquaint themselves with the impact early cosmology has had on medicine. Awareness of this linkage can help us better understand not only past but present-day medicine.

From Antiquity, many healers have been astronomer-physicians, including such thinkers as Pythagoras, Hippocrates, Empedocles, and Eudoxus. Some notables, such as Aristotle, Manilius, Ptolemy, Firmicus, Augustine of Hippo, Albertus Magnus, and a host of others, though not trained in medicine, tried their hand at healing, astronomy and/or astrology. It was not uncommon for past scholars (polymaths) to be involved in many intellectual pursuits. Hippocrates (or his disciples) was convinced that knowledge of astronomy, including meteorology, was essential to the practice of medicine:

> For knowing the changes of the seasons, and the risings and settings of the stars, with the circumstances of each of these phenomena, he (the physician) will know beforehand the nature of the year that is coming, through these considerations and by learning the times beforehand, he will have full knowledge of each particular case (patient), will succeed best in securing health, and will achieve the greatest triumphs in the practice of his art. If it be thought that all this belongs to meteorology, he will find out, on second thought, that the contribution of astronomy to medicine is not a very small one but a very great one, indeed. [4]

From these early times to the present, the fancied or real impact of astronomy on health has persisted in a continuous parade of practitioners of both sciences. The first purpose of this book is to establish, in a complete and organized manner, how cosmology, astronomy and universal harmony have provided the theoretical foundations for the practice of medicine in Antiquity and the Middle Ages. Although much has been written about ancient and medieval medicine, including its basic theoretical foundations, until now no thoroughgoing, coherent exegesis of this area of pre-modern medicine has been attempted. It will be demonstrated, using primary sources, that the cosmology of the ancients provides not only the theoretical basis for the etiology of disease but also the rationale for its treatment. Material from prehistory is presented including mythical, philosophical, and historical evidence, to support the thesis that universal harmony, as found in the cosmology of the ancients, formed the basis for medical practice well into the nineteenth century.

In the twentieth century, the well-known English astrophysicist, Fred Hoyle, perpetuated this tradition in *Diseases from Space*. In this treatise Hoyle presents arguments, which he thought support the idea that viruses and bacteria come from outer space.

> In *Diseases from Space*, we shall be presenting arguments and facts, which support the idea that viruses and bacteria responsible for the infectious diseases of plants and animals arrive at the Earth from space.

Hoyle hypothesizes that comets are the home breeding ground for these viruses and bacteria, and that, when Earth passes through the remnants of a comet, our atmosphere and ultimately the creatures living on Earth, are exposed to the pathogens responsible for epidemic diseases such as influenza. As fanciful and incredible Hoyle's thesis may be, it is a holdover from the early Enlightenment when Isaac Newton and Edmund Halley, among others, believed that comets were the cause of many human disasters. We now know this is not the case. While *Diseases from Space* reads like the play, *The Mouse Trap*, which under Hoyle's direction, ends with a hung jury, the saga that led to modern medicine plays like a documentary film that is more fascinating than the most fanciful novel. As fascinating as space medicine is, it is no more exciting than the journey that brought us to the practice of modern medicine. This book for the first time relates this saga of healing.

The first two parts of this book show that the four elements of earth, water, air and fire as outlined by Empedocles in the fifth century B.C.E., are the basic components of sublunary beings. Empedocles tied these four elements to the four qualities of hot, cold, wet and dry, which in turn are connected to the four humors: blood, phlegm, yellow and black bile and thence to the four temperaments associated with the four humors: sanguine, phlegmatic, cholic and melancholic. In turn, all these relationships can be tied to the ancient and medieval concepts of disease etiology, diagnosis, treatment and prognosis. This scheme provides a rational connection between the heavens and human health; all of which is developed in a clear and logical way so the reader can understand why the ancients and medievals believed so fervently in the medicine of their day. How these ideas evolved over the centuries is covered, utilizing works from various early medical writers and practitioners.

The second purpose of the book flows from the first, which is to explain the puzzling persistence of a medical system that clearly did not work and yet continued to be followed for so many centuries. The adherence to "authority," which was so ingrained in ancient and medieval cultures, along with the hierarchical authority of the medieval Church are offered as two (of several) reasons for the slavish adherence to the principles of ancient medicine. Pervasive insecurity, as found in the Middle Ages, also played a role in the persistence of ancient medical theory. Additionally, true empiricism was unknown in early medicine. Until Roger Bacon and later Francis Bacon, finally developed a better understanding of the scientific method, progress in any of the sciences was not possible. All science up to this point had been based on anecdotal observations which, along with speculative reasoning, were considered an adequate basis for "science." The empirical method took centuries to develop. The transition from medieval to modern medicine is reviewed to demonstrate how the chains of medieval medicine were finally broken. It was this process of change that, in the end, undermined the factors responsible for the long life of Galenic medicine.

Notes

1. Kramer, S. N. 1959. *History Begins at Sumer* (Garden City, NY: Doubleday) chapters 10 and 13.
2. Tester, S. J. 1999. *A History of Western Astrology* (Rochester, NY: Bondell Press).
3. Aristotle. 1952. *Aristotle's Metaphysics*, trans. R. Hope (New York: Columbia University Press).
4. Hippocrates. 1923. *Writings*, vol. I-IV, "Water, Air, Places," Loeb Classics, trans. W.H. S. Jones (London: Harvard University Press).
5. Crowe, M. J. 1990. *Theories of the World from Antiquity to the Copernican Revolution* (New York: Dover).
6. Debus, A. G. 1970. *Harvey and Fludd: The Irrational Factor in the Rational Science of the Seventeenth Century*," Journal of the History of Biology, 3, 81
7. Edelstein, L. 1967. *Ancient Medicine*, ed. O. Temkin and C. L. Temkin (Baltimore, MD: Johns Hopkins University Press).
8. Guthrie, K. S. 1987. *The Pythagorean Source Book and Library* (Grand Rapids, MI): Phanes Press.
9. Lambridis, H. 1976. *Empedocles* (University: University of Alabama Press).
10. Lindberg, D. C. 1978. *Science in the Middle Ages* (Chicago: University of Chicago Press).
11. Neugebauer, O. and van Hoesen, H. B. 1959. *Greek Horoscopes* (Philadelphia: American Philosophical Society).
12. Neugebauer, O. 1969. *The Exact Sciences in Antiquity* (New York: Dover).
13. Rawcliffe, C. 1999. *Medicine and Society in Later Medieval England* (London: Sandpiper).
14. Siraisi, N. G. 1990. *Medieval and Renaissance Medicine* (Chicago: University of Chicago Press).
15. Hoyle, F. 1979. *Diseases from Space* (New York: Harper & Row).

Part 1
The Beginnings

1

Prehistory

Ancient Artifacts

Little is known about the astronomy-medicine connection before recorded history but some clues can be pieced together to help light this dark, primitive period.[1] Haggard has suggested the presence of "medicine men" among the Cro-Magnon tribes that lived 25,000 years ago. This idea is based on cave paintings from southwest France.

Whether this is a correct interpretation of this cave art and whether these "doctors" sought the aid of the stars in their healing may never be known. A prehistoric ivory figure may lend some credence to the claim that there was a very early connection between medicine and the stars.[2] It is hypothesized that this ivory carving is of the constellation Orion and the notches engraved on it indicate it was used to determine a pregnant woman's due date. Again, this is a postulate that is hard to prove.

Stone Circles

Some evidence to support such claims, however, may come from the stone circles of England[3] and North America.[4] Mên-an-Tol[5] is one such site. This stone circle dates from around 2000 B.C.E. and the name in Cornish means stone hole. Many of these structures are known and each site consists of several stones, at least one of which is upright with a hole large enough for an adult to pass through it.

At Mên-an-Tol the stone is four feet high and the orientation of the associated stones is NW-SE, suggesting, as with Stonehenge and other northern European stone circles, an astronomical arrangement.[6] This geometry has been interpreted by many scholars as indicating a primitive astronomical observatory that locates the rising of the Sun at the summer solstice as well as other solar alignments of agricultural and religious significance. Moon positions, the nineteen-year Moon-solar cycle and even predictions of lunar eclipses[7] have been offered as observational functions for these stone groupings.

3

The circles marked sunrise for both May Day and the beginning of August, along with the times of sunset for the first day of February and November. These times were the four great pagan "quarter-day" festivals. The Moon position may also have been aligned with the stones. Mên-an-Tol is of interest because it may have medical as well as astronomical significance. It is speculated that sick children were passed through the stone hole at certain seasons of the Moon. Various religious as well as eschatological purposes have been offered for the stones' function. The medical use is most credible because even during the Victorian period, sick children were passed through the stone hole nine times in a healing ritual that may have persisted over the centuries, passed on from generation to generation. The use of various types of stones for healing purposes has a long history.[8] Healing stones, as we shall see, were used in the Middle Ages along with herbs for therapeutic purposes. Even today "stones" in the form of calcium carbonate and calamine are used to treat osteoporosis and pruritic (itchy) rashes!

Medicine Wheels

In North America, so-called "Medicine Wheels" have been discovered that appear to have astronomical significance.[9] These consist of stone wheels (circles) with radiating spokes spread out on the ground. They are found throughout the eastern edge of the Rocky Mountains in the United States and Canada. There are about fifty of these "medicine wheels." Their purpose is unknown but seems to relate to social or religious rituals. The name Medicine Wheel is more recent in origin and may not necessarily indicate a medical use for these structures, though they could have been used for ritual healing in the distant past. They are made from local rocks laid out on the ground in simple patterns, ranging in size from six to several hundred feet in diameter. The stones radiate from a central hub to an outer circle of stones and, viewed from above, look like a sun symbol. Some have large central cairns containing as much as 100 tons of rock. Many of these wheels have a NE-SW orientation aligned with the summer solstice. Certain Native American ceremonies were associated with the summer solstice, possibly related to agricultural interests.

The Big Horn Medicine Wheel, located near Sheraton, Wyoming, is the best known of these stone circles and shows the most definite astronomical alignments. It has twenty-eight spokes. A line drawn from the southwest cairn, which is outside the stone circle, through the central

Figure 1.1

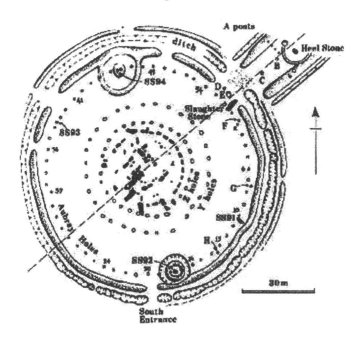

Here is shown a schematic of Stonehenge with its stone circle and "ditch and mound" earthen circle in which water may collect. In addition, there is depicted the orientation of the circle, which points directly at the Sun at the precise moment of the summer solstice.

cairn, lies within 0.2° of the rising Sun at the summer solstice. Another southeast cairn aligned with the central cairn marks the summer solstice sunset. The probability that these are chance alignments is estimated to be about one in 4,000. Three of the cairns are arranged to mark the heliacal risings of the stars Aldebaran, Rigel and Sirius. Between 1400 and 1700 c.e., Aldebaran marked the time of the summer solstice. Rigel rose heliacally 28 days after Aldebaran and Sirius rose heliacally twenty-eight days after Rigel. Twenty-eight was a favorite number among the Indians of North America and along with the 28 spokes in the wheel, suggests a lunar/stellar connection. These findings would fit with an astronomical use for the Medicine Wheels. Whether they were used as healing sites, as their modern name suggests, may never be known, though such associations are found in other ancient cultures. It is probable that the Medicine Wheels developed independently of the European stone circles.

Figure 1.2
Medicine Wheel in Big Horn Mountains

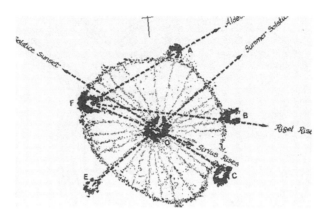

The Druids

The Druids bridge the boundary between prehistory and history, allowing a glimpse into the dim, distant past. They are a mysterious group whose exact identity and origins are shrouded in a historical haze. Some authors portray them as savage seers who performed human sacrifices and used ill-gotten entrails to foretell the future. Ellis suggests that they were more likely a

> ...Caste incorporating all the learned professions. This caste not only consisted of those who had a religious function but also consisted of philosophers, judges, teachers, historians, poets, musicians, physicians, astronomers, prophets and political advisers or counselors. [10]

Among the ancient Romans, Strabo, Julius Caesar, Diodorus Siculus, Cicero, Pliny the Elder, and Tacitus all praise the Druids for their knowledge of astronomy.[11] This last author further notes that Pomponius Mela claims that the "Druids knew the size and shape of the world, the movement of the heavens and of the stars, as well as the lunar effect on the tides and the cause of the midnight Sun." Hippolytus believed that the Druids could foretell certain heavenly events by Pythagorean calculations. Pliny reports that the Druids watched the course of the Moon in order to determine the proper time to cut mistletoe—thus suggesting a link between their function as astronomers and physicians. Mistletoe was highly prized by the Druids for both religious and medicinal purposes. Pliny[12] tells of the magical healing powers attributed to this plant by the Druids.

Druids appear as healers in many Irish and Welsh tales.[13] Pliny claims that the name, "Druid" is derived from the Greek word for oak (δρυζ)). The oak tree, along with the mistletoe that grew upon it, was held sacred by the Druids.

> They believed that anything growing on oak-trees is sent by heaven. The mistletoe was collected on the sixth day of the Moon. Then greeting the Moon with the phrase that in their own language means healing all things…. They think that mistletoe given in a drink renders any barren animals fertile and is an antidote for all poisons.

This passage from Pliny gives clear evidence that the Druids as priest-physicians utilized astronomy in their healing art. Medicine was mixed with astronomy—a practice common in Antiquity. Pliny's portrayal of the Druids may be our clearest evidence of the influence of astronomy on medicine in prehistory.

Healing and Health Hazards in the Heavens

The origin of star names is largely lost in prehistory. Many of the stars bear Arabic names, some coming from the early Babylonians or Arabic tribes, but most were borrowed by Arabs of the early Middle Ages from Greek or Latin sources. Very early on, only individual stars were named; later asterisms (star groupings) were identified, often based on common objects found in daily life. These included anatomical parts such as eyes, arms, legs, thorax, abdomen, as well as animals (Leo the Lion) and mythical figures (Orion the Hunter).

Asclepius the Healer

Aratus of Soloi (c. 315 - 245 B.C.E.) was one of the first and most famous commentators on stars and constellations. *Phenomena*,[14] written about 270 B.C.E., was used by Hipparchus in his second century B.C.E. astronomical writings. For centuries astronomers relied on this work in observing the skies. Aratus saw in the heavens the writings of God that were given to humans for their benefit which included a healthier life. Aratus describes Ophiuchos as the Serpent-Holder with

> "Both hands grip [ping] the Serpent that coils around his waist, and with feet firmly planted he crushed the monstrous Scorpion, one foot on his eyes and one on the thorax as he stands upright."[15]

Ophiuchus has been portrayed as the "serpent charmer"; one who can cure the bites of poisonous snakes.[16] This mythical person is generally identified with Asclepius who, from Greek times, has been portrayed as the god of medicine. Asclepius was said to be the son of Apollo, one of the Olympian gods also associated with medicine. Coronis, the mother of Asclepius, had been unfaithful to Apollo while pregnant with Apollo's child. For this act of impiety, she was sentenced to death by Apollo. However, while on her funeral pyre, remorsefully, he snatched the future god of medicine from the flames, presumably by performing a caesarean section. The newborn was to become the most famous physician of mythology. Asclepius is usually associated with a snake and the myths of Asclepius include his healing of Glaucus, son of Minos, the king of Crete.[17] Glaucus had, in fact, already died. King Minos put Asclepius in prison and while pondering how to restore Glaucus to life, Asclepius observed a snake crawling up his staff. Without hesitation, he killed it. Later another snake came out of the ground carrying an herb in its mouth and proceeded to place it on the head of the dead reptile, which immediately came to life. Using the same herb, Asclepius proceeded to restore Glaucus to life. This is one explanation for the origin of the caduceus as a symbol of healing. Similar myths abound in ancient Greek literature, the most famous concerning Hippolytus, who died in a chariot accident.[18] Asclepius restored him to life using the serpent's herb. This medical miracle, however, caused problems with the gods.

> Clymenus and Clotho grieved, that life's broken thread should be re-spun, he that his kingdom's rights should be infringed. [19]

Jupiter in anger killed Asclepius with a thunderbolt. Apollo, saddened by the loss of his son, raised him into the sky as a god. Thus, Asclepius remains forever as healer in the heavens.

Centaurus, the Centaur (half man and half horse) was identified by Eratosthenes as Χείρων Chiron who was assigned by Apollo to mentor Asclepius in the medical arts.[20] This astronomical association between Chiron, the medical teacher, and Ophiuchus, the healer, has persisted through the centuries. Apollo and Diana had taught Chiron astronomy and medicine as well as music and botany—the latter two having value in the healing arts, as we shall see later. Chiron has made his presence known even in modern astronomy. Kowal et al.[21] first described a new class of celestial objects, the Centaur population; objects with perihelia beyond Jupiter but with semi-major axes smaller than Neptune's. Their orbits are unstable as a result of the perturbations induced by the giant planet's gravitational pull and are in dynamic transition from the trans-Neptunian Kuiper belt to the inner solar system.[22] Chiron was the mythical name applied to the first of this class of astronomical objects. Thus, Chiron, the medical "professor" of Antiquity continues to attract interest today.

Healthy and Unhealthy Stars

There are many other healing aspects to the celestial sphere. The horn of Monoceros,[23] the unicorn, was thought to possess medicinal qualities and, as a result, ground-up cattle horns were fraudulently sold as a medicament in the Middle Ages.[24] Pindar (c. 522-443 B.C.E.) suggests that Aquarius the Water Bearer symbolizes the life-giving waters of the Nile. Some claim that Aquarius brought the Nile floods when the Sun entered this constellation (as it did 15,000 years ago), bringing a bountiful harvest and healthy food to the Egyptians.[25] Arcturus, Hippocrates claims, might bring a dry season and a poor crop causing malnutrition.[26] Cancer the Crab has no mythological relationship to our modern day neoplasms but was a perceived health hazard, the story is told that Cancer pinched Hercules' toes during his battle with the Hydra and in response the strong man crushed Cancer, destroying the dangerous crustacean as Ophiuchus had done to Scorpio.[27] Cancer was thought to "reign over" afflictions of the human breast and stomach. Doctor Ben Johnson, the English writer, referred to "fevers of the Crab," thus making a connection between this constellation and febrile illnesses.[28] Various stars in Cancer were tied to blindness and the clavicle (collar bone). Canis Major and especially its alpha star, Sirius, have a rich mythical history. In Egypt, Sirius was associated with the fertile flooding of the Nile. This star also had some negative connotations, causing "fevers, plague and death."[29] Capricornus is portrayed as the nurse of young Apollo, the god of medicine.[30] In the Middle Ages, this constellation was worn as an amulet—a kind of "astral defensive armor" against a variety of maladies.[31] Crux the Cross was originally part of Centaurus (Chiron) whose knowledge of medicine has already been discussed.[32]

Cygnus the Swan has been associated with Orpheus and his lyre (Lyra). Orpheus was able to bring his wife Eurydice nearly back to life by charming the god of the underworld, Hades, with his music.[33] Unfortunately, Orpheus, who had been warned against looking back as he left the underworld, did so, losing his wife forever to the adamantine walls of Hell. As we shall see, Pythagoras, the astronomer and mathematician (and healer), along with Orpheus, believed in the healing value of music and harmony. Delphinus the Dolphin in some myths has acted as a pilot guiding Bacchus safely across the seas, thus averting any bodily injuries on the way,[34] And there are several health hazards in the sky that Hercules faced in his labors, including Draco the Dragon, Leo the Lion, and Hydra, as well as pesky Cancer the Crab and Scorpio the Scorpion.

Asclepius healed Hercules wounds after one of his battles. Gemini, the Twins were said to have power over health of the hands, arms and shoulders.[35] The great plague of London (1665-1666) was blamed on Gemini. Ancient physicians believed that when the Sun was in Leo the Lion, normally helpful medicines could become poisons to their patients.[36] Even a bath in this setting might be lethal. Lupus the Wolf was considered the "Beast of Death" although some saw the asterism as a Centaur, possibly Chiron, teacher of Asclepius.[37] Lyra the Lyre was viewed by some Ancients as a vulture and thus symbolic of death.[38]

In Egypt, Orion the Hunter had many after-life associations but in terms of health hazards, he is connected to Scorpio the Scorpion because he was said to have died of the bite of this poisonous arachnid and ever since hides under the western horizon when Scorpio rises in the east.[39] Pavo the Peacock is one of Bayer's later-named twelve constellations, and this bird is a symbol of immortality.[40] The mythical hero Perseus killed the Medusa and used her snake-ridden head to turn Cetus the Sea Monster into stone, thereby saving the fair maiden Andromeda. The constellation Phoenix is also one of Bayer's newer stellar figures and, as with the Phoenix itself, represents the cycle of death and rebirth and, as it was for the Egyptians, is symbolic of immortality.[41] Pliny suggests that the appearance of a comet in Pisces the Fishes was the source of pestilence.[42]

Sagittarius the Archer is a centaur like Chiron, depicted as aiming his arrow at Scorpio's heart (Antares) and protecting against the sting of the scorpion.[43] Pliny, likewise, predicted a plague of reptiles and insects if a comet appeared in Scorpio.[44] The Pleiades are depicted as nursing the young Zeus with ambrosia.[45] And both the Milky Way and later the Magellanic Clouds were thought of as sources of nurturing milk for the gods. The word "galaxy" is derived from the Greek for milk.

Thus, the heavens are rich with references to health and health hazards. Health was a constant concern for the Ancients. Astronomy and medicine were ever present in their lives and the association of heaven and health could hardly be avoided. People were afflicted by a host of ailments and injuries, most of which could not be treated. There was no light pollution and the stars sparkled brilliantly every clear night. The stars appeared so close it seemed that one could reach up and touch them. No wonder the heavens became involved in the lives and health of the Ancients. As we shall see, the early Greeks viewed the stars as divine, living beings that were not only physically above the world in which these people lived and died, but also as divine beings held sway over every aspect of their lives. The mythical medicine of the world above was very real to the healer and astronomer of ancient Greece. Recourse to the stars (and planets) was often all the physician had to guide him in diagnosis, therapy and prognosis for his languishing patient.

Notes

1. Haggard, H. W. 1962. *The Doctor in History* (Freeport, NY: Books for Libraries Press), p. 6.
2. Rappenglück, M. 2003. "Fertile Theory," *Science*, 299: 817.
3. Cooke, I. 1987. *Mermaid to Merrymaid: Journey to the Stones* (Over Wallop, UK: BAS Printers).
4. Eddy, J. A. 1978. *In Search of Ancient Astronomy*, ed. E. C. Krupp (New York: McGraw-Hill).
5. Cooke, I. 1987, *Mermaid*, p. 43.
6. Castleden, R. 1987. *The Stonehenge People* (New York: Routledge & Kegan Paul), pp. 128-132.
7. Challener, S. 2000. 195th AAS meeting, #92.01.
8. Best, M.R. and Brightman, F.H. 1999. *The Book of Secrets of Albertus Magnus* (York Beach, ME: Samuel Weiser).
9. Eddy, J. A. 1978, *Ancient Astronomy*, p. 159.
10. Ellis, P. B. 1994. *The Druids* (New York: William B. Erdmans), p. 14.
11. Ibid., p. 229.
12. Pliny. 1991. *Natural History: A Selection*, trans. J. Healy (New York: Penguin), p. 216.
13. Ellis. 1994, *Druids*, p. 213.
14. Aratus. 1983. *Phaenomena* (Berkeley, CA: North Atlantic Books).
15. Ibid., p. 4.
16. Ibid., p. 298.
17. Mayerson, P. 1971. *Classical Mythology in Literature, Art and Music* (New York: John Wiley & Sons), p. 132.
18. Edelstein, E. and Edelstein, L. 1998. *Asclepius: Collection and Interpretation of the Testimonies* (Baltimore, MD: Johns Hopkins University Press), pp. 42-43.
19. Atropos, Clotho and Lachesis were the mythological Fates. Atropos carries the shears and cuts the thread of life, Clotho has the spindle and spins the thread of life while Lachesis holds the globe or scroll that determines the length of life. Interfering with the Fates was an act of impiety.
20. Allen, R. H. 1963. *Star Names*, pp. 148-149.
21. Koval, C. T. 1979, "The Discovery and Orbit of (2060) Chiron, IAUS," *Dynamics of the Solar System*, 81:245.
22. Fernandez, Y. R. et al. 2002, "Thermal Properties of Centaurs Asbolus and Chiron," *Astronomical Journal*, 123, 1050. Perturbations are disturbances in the orbit of a celestial object caused by the gravitational pull of both Jupiter and Neptune. Eventually, Chiron (2060) will be pulled closer to the Sun.
23. Monoceros is a constellation near Orion.
24. Haggard, H. W. 1962, *Doctor*, p. 28.
25. Allen, R. H. 1963, *Star Names*, p. 47.
26. Ibid., p. 100.

27.   Ibid., p. 107.
28.   Ibid., p. 110.
29.   Ibid., p. 125.
30.   Ibid., p. 135.
31.   Ibid., p. 137.
32.   Ibid., p. 184.
33.   Ibid., p. 193.
34.   Ibid., p. 199.
35.   Ibid., p. 228.
36.   Ibid., p. 253.
37.   Ibid., p. 278.
38.   Ibid., p. 286.
39.   Ibid., p. 303.
40.   Ibid., p. 321.
41.   Ibid., p. 331.
42.   Ibid., p.340.
43.   Ibid., p. 352.
44.   Ibid., p. 364.
45.   Ibid., p. 395.

2

The Ancients

The Egyptians

There is debate as to whether the Babylonians or Egyptians were the first true astronomers,[1] but there is little doubt concerning the Egyptians' medical skills.[2] Homer is quoted as saying that the doctors of Egypt "are skilled beyond all men." The Persian kings of antiquity, Cyrus and Darius, both used Egyptian physicians. The Edwin Smith and Ebers Papyri provide evidence of ancient Egyptians studying both surgery and medicine.[3] This medical education often took place at the various temples where herbal gardens were kept and physicians practiced. The temple priests were both astronomers and physicians. Included in the medical papyri are herbal therapies, prayers, chants and spells. Incantations were commonly accepted "medical" therapies used by both physicians and temple priests.

The sophistication of ancient Egyptian astronomy is uncertain but there is increasing evidence that they aligned the great pyramids at Giza with Sirius and astronomy was used for agricultural purposes. The heliacal rising of Sirius (4,000 years ago) was in June and coincided with flooding of the Nile, which provided irrigation for the wheat crop.[4,5] The Egyptians are given credit for the 365-day, twelve-month calendrical year. In the Babylonian, Greek, and Roman cultures, a lunar calendar was used. Part of the difficulty in assessing the Egyptians' astronomical knowledge is their unwillingness to allow foreigners access to their "secret wisdom." Much of the astronomical data used by the Egyptians involved religious ritual. Temple priests were responsible for prayer times and a priest would stay up throughout the night tracking star movements in order to properly time these prayer periods. In order to predict the proper time for these rituals, the priest needed accurate knowledge of the skies. A compelling example of the astronomer-physician is Imhotep, a legendary figure in Egyptian history, who was the architect responsible for the "Step Pyramids" at Saqqara.[6] According to I. E. S. Edwards in *The Pyramids of Egypt,* Imhotep, in addition to being one of the first architects, was also a priest, magician, astronomer and father of medicine.[7] The Greeks identified him with Asclepius, their god of medicine.

There seems little doubt that both astronomy and medicine were disciplines found in the priestly repertoire and that their astronomy was mirrored in their medicine. As Johnson[8] says, "Observational astronomy which kept the calendar up to date was, like medicine, a priestly profession." Since Imhotep probably lived in the fourth or third millennium B.C.E., it appears that, as with the Sumerians and Druids, the astronomy-medicine connection dates to the very early times of recorded history and likely began in prehistory.

The Greeks

Pythagoras

Pythagoras (c. 580-c. 500 B.C.E.) was one of the most influential Greek philosophers and mathematicians. He was also a healer and astronomer.[9] His world-order was based on numbers, which for Pythagoras possessed a reality of their own. According to Photus (820-891 B.C.E.), "It was Pythagoras who first called heaven *kosmos* because it is perfect, and "adorned" with infinite beauty and living beings." [10] He proposed an undifferentiated unity out of which the world-order or cosmos emerged. For Pythagoras, cosmos means an "ornamented order" or beautiful Universe. From this follows his concept of harmony and the fundamental role music plays in the world system. Although the concept of harmony may have developed earlier, it was Pythagoras who made it a defined cosmological system. Pythagoras developed a system of "opposites." These sets of opposites arose out of the "unity" through a process unexplained by the Pythagoreans. Two opposites then reunite to generate life. Subsequently, this world of opposites is articulated more fully by Aristotle[11] in the *Metaphysics*. These opposites include: limited-unlimited, odd-even, one-plurality, etc. Aristotle asserts that in the Pythagorean system everything is made up of numbers but Aristotle views this as only partially true. For Pythagoras, everything is composed of the "elements" of numbers which are the opposing principles described above. According to Aristotle, Pythagoras replaced the four elements with numbers as the basic building blocks of the sublunary physical world.[12] At any rate, this system is speculative and not observable, that is, non-empirical.[13]

In terms of Pythagoras' medicine, it is known that he was trained as a healer by the Egyptians and most likely learned his astronomy from them as well. Pythagoras had several biographers from whom much can be determined about his life. Though he was born on the Mediterranean island of Samos, historians agree that he spent twenty-two years studying in the temples of Egypt.[14] He was ultimately initiated into "all the mysteries of the gods " according to Iamblicus, one of his biographers.[15] He is thought to have been the first foreigner to be so honored. That Pythagoras was acquainted with medicine is supported by the fact that he was described by later generations as the son of Apollo, the god of both medicine and music. According to Porphyry, another of his biographers, when Pherecydes, an early teacher of Pythagoras, fell ill in Delos, Pythagoras traveled there from Croton, in southern Italy, to "attend him until he died."[16] In addition, Pythagoras and his school espoused a number of health related concepts. One of his basic tenets was that of "purification" of both the body and soul. He advocated abstinence from wine and meat. He is quoted by Porphyry[17] as having said:

> We ought to the best of our ability avoid, and even with fire and sword, eradicate from the body, sickness; from the soul, ignorance; from the belly, luxury; from a city, sedition; from a family, discord; and from all things, excess.

Porphyry further notes that, "He soothed the passions of the soul and body by rhythms, songs and incantations. He would calm himself every morning by singing, dancing and playing the lyre, thereby soothing his mind and conferring on the body agility and health." This emphasis on music therapy is consistent with his concept of universal harmony and he is credited with being the father of this branch of medicine. That he functioned as a healer is further supported by Porphyry[18] who notes, that if friends, "were sick, he nursed them; if they were afflicted in the mind, he solaced them, some by incantations and magic charms, some by music." The use of incantations is further evidence of the medical training received in the temples of Egypt, since they were used extensively by the temple priests. Porphyry also confirms that Pythagoras nursed his former teacher, Pherecydes, while he was dying.[19]

Pythagoras saw the cosmos and the body as a harmonious unity. Songs soothed the soul and body but there were also songs in the heavens. He claimed that we did not hear these cosmic chords because we were so used to them but they were nonetheless there. This connectedness of body and cosmos was articulated in his concepts of macrocosm and microcosm. Photus states:[20]

> Pythagoras said that man was a microcosm, which means a compendium of the Universe...he is constituted by the four elements...he contains all the powers of the cosmos. For the Universe contains God, the four elements, animals and plants. All these powers are contained in man. He has reason, which is a divine power; he has the nature of the elements; and the powers of moving, growing and reproduction.

Pythagoras was the first to propose the macrocosm-microcosm connection. This was ultimately the basis for the influences of the heavens on health. As is the case with Hippocrates, it is important to understand that not all that is Pythagorean was from Pythagoras himself, but developed out of his school at Croton in southern Italy. In a real sense, Pythagoras was Father of Medical Theory. He called the Universe Cosmos (order), defined the Universe as based on harmony, believed all objects in the heavens produced music, and was the first to discover the mathematical basis of harmonic theory. This, along with the macro-microcosm connection between the heavens and each individual human, provided the fundamental basis of medicine for the next 2,400 years. All medical theory that followed simply elaborated on Pythagoras' system.

The Greeks after Pythagoras

Early Greek astronomy and medicine were highly speculative sciences. They were considered subdivisions of "natural philosophy" and what seemed rational and logical to the Greeks was held to be true, often in spite of empirical evidence to the contrary. They were said to have "tried to explain nature while shutting their eyes"[21] Alcmaeon of Croton, an early Greek physician and philosopher, lived in the sixth century B.C.E. He is said to have been the founder of empirical psychology and was also the first to propose that health was a state of balance of opposites within the body and, conversely, diseases the excess or deficiency of one or more of these opposites.[22] Alcmaeon began a theoretical trend that was to be taken up later by Hippocrates, Aristotle and Galen. As we shall see, the opposites became hot and cold, wet and dry. Alcmaeon, however, posited a host of contraries including black and white, sweet and bitter, good and evil, small and great, and so on.[23] The idea of contraries was thus established as a medical theme.

Philolaus (c.475 B.C.E.) appears to have been the first to offer an imbalance of bile, blood, or phlegm as the cause of disease. These humors were to occupy medical theory until the modern period. Empedocles[24] (c. 490-430 B.C.E.), a "distinguished physician" as well as a cosmologist, believed that the cosmos was in a perpetual cycle, continually destroyed and reformed.[25] He is generally credited with developing the concept of the four elements: earth, water, air, and fire. Empedocles appears to have added "earth" to the other three elements which had been offered by earlier philosophers as constituents of the physical world. This contribution to cosmology was very important for the medical concepts that were to become the cornerstone of disease theory and therapy in both Antiquity and the Middle Ages. The qualities, humors, and elements were to become the essential features of medieval medicine.

Hippocrates

Hippocrates (c.460-c. 377 B.C.E.) is known as the first empirical medical practitioner. Up to his time much of medical theory consisted of conjecture and "hypotheses," which he and his school denounced as unsatisfactory because this approach relied more on speculation and superstition than observation and experience.[26] He also denied the "divine" as a cause of disease. God did not create disease in humans. For Hippocrates (and his followers) sickness depended on "environment" and human "constituents." Hippocrates viewed environment as consisting of the "spheres" of the Universe. These spheres included the heavens (composed of ether) and the sublunary region (derived from earth, water, air and fire). Disease and health were intertwined with the world above and about us and the cause of disease was to be found not only in the workings of the body but in the heavens—in the atmosphere and climate which were determined by the heavenly spheres. It was in "Nature" that diseases developed and in "Nature" that cures were to be found. All the physician could do was to allow Nature a chance to work. The remedies offered in his *Regimens in Acute Disease*[27] include:

1.Purgatives and emetics.
2. Fomentations (poultices and warm compresses) and baths.
3. Barley-water and barley gruel.
4. Wine.
5. Hydromel (honey and water) and oxymel (honey and vinegar).
6. Venesection (bloodletting).
7. Rest and a soothing environment.

These were simple remedies which offer some medicinal value in today's terms but mainly allow Nature to work its cures. As the medieval saying has it, *Medicus curat, Natura sanat:* Doctors treat and Nature cures. Hippocrates, states unequivocally in *Air, Water, Places:*[28]

> The contribution of astronomy to medicine is not a very small one but a very great one, indeed,....(knowledge) of the rising and setting of stars (which include the planets)....and of the seasons, the winds, the Moon, Sun and stars will allow the physician to, succeed best in securing health, and will achieve the greatest triumphs in the practice of his art.

Knowing the diseases that a season or particular wind might bring was essential to the practice of medicine. Whether the winds are hot or cold, southerly or northerly, allows the physician to predict future diseases. Certain winds may bring plagues. Water and soil play a role in health as does the atmosphere. Winter brings certain disease such as dysentery, "ague" (chills, fever, and sweats), asthma and even hemorrhoids, according to Hippocrates. Epilepsy was labeled the "sacred disease" because it was thought to be caused by the heavens. Whether this meant a divine cause or heavenly influences is not certain but it is likely the latter, since Hippocrates dismissed divine causes of disease. Catarrhs (inflammation of the nose, throat and chest) occurred, "when the Sun suddenly strikes the patient's head." On the other hand, Hippocrates maintains that, "Those that lie toward the rising of the Sun are likely to be healthier.... For the Sun shining down upon them when it rises, purifies them." This purification process may be derived from earlier Pythagorean teachings.[29] By contrast, "Those that lie toward the setting of the Sun....the hot winds and the cold north winds blow past them—these cities must have a most unhealthy situation." Hippocrates saw similar effects in the clouds, rain, winds and stars.[30]

> If at the rising of the Dog Star (Sirius) stormy rain occurs and the Etesian winds (prevailing northerly summer winds of the Mediterranean) blow there is hope that the distempers will cease and the autumn will be healthy.

The Ancients were aware that the Sun influenced health. They knew that certain seasons were associated with specific diseases just as such associations are known today. They were not, however, aware of bacterial or viral diseases and so it was logical to assign causation to concomitants of disease, even though correlation does not necessarily imply causation. This was not astrological medicine in the true sense, as we shall see when studying the Romans later, but rather an attempt to make sense out of the pathology at hand.

The Humors

The four elements (earth, water, air, and fire) and the four qualities of the body (hot, cold, wet, and dry) were all essential features of ancient and medieval medicine. Anaximander (611-547 B.C.E.), according to

Hippocrates,[31] may have proposed the concept of "opposites" (though Philolaus and Pythagoras, had a hand in developing these ideas as well). Later thinkers expanded on the role of the four qualities. In *Ancient Medicine*[32] Hippocrates refers to the qualities as "powers."[33] These powers, however, were secondary to the four humors that formed the final facet of the cause and cure of diseases. The four humors were part of both the Hippocratic school and Galen's scheme of diseases and these two ideologues sculpted the form medicine was to take through the Middle Ages. It was not until the Enlightenment that this paradigm of medical care was to be dethroned.

The four humors were phlegm, blood, yellow bile, and black bile.[34] These humors were first clearly defined in the *Nature of Man*, thought by some to have been written by Hippocrates, though Aristotle attributes this treatise to Polybus, the son-in-law of Hippocrates.[35]

Why these four fluids became the "backbone" of medicine is uncertain. Fluids are obviously essential to life and this may have played a role in choosing these as essential fluids. Phlegm was produced in excess with many respiratory diseases, blood was clearly necessary to life and both yellow and black bile were often seen in vomitus.[36]

There are many variations on humoral theory but, in essence, they were thought to account for both personality and disease. The four personalities were the phlegmatic, sanguine, cholic and melancholic depending on the predominant humor in a given individual. The phlegmatic person was laid back and relaxed; the sanguine animated, gregarious and humorous; the cholic, ill tempered and flammable; and the melancholic lugubrious and moody. Either an excess or deficiency of a humor accounted for disease. The idea of therapy was to restore the balance in the body of the unbalanced humor(s). As will be more fully outlined when dealing with Aristotle, the humors, powers, and elements were paired in various ways to explain diseases and their remedies. The point to be noted here is that the heavens influence these elements, powers and humors and, thus are involved in health and disease. We shall see later how this scheme was more fully formulated.

Plato

Plato (c.427-347 B.C.E) was neither a physician nor an observational astronomer. His cosmology was strictly speculative and based, in part, on Pythagorean concepts. His postulates, however, were to influence both astronomy and medicine for centuries to come. Plato's approach to any subject was philosophical and speculative. Empirical endeavors were foreign to his worldview. For Plato the physical world was merely a shadowy reflection of "Ideas" or "Forms" that existed outside our world of perception and represented the "real" world. These Ideas were the only truly existent and absolute entities; everything else was but a faint, imperfect copy. The Forms are the only true objects of philosophical inquiry.[37] The study of the physical world would ultimately lead to error and a failed paradigm of the world. This highly speculative approach may have delayed the advance of the scientific method for many hundreds of years, in spite of Aristotle's (student of Plato) subsequent empirical orientation. Platonism held sway until Aristotle was rediscovered in the twelfth century when Arabic copies of his works became available.

Plato's cosmology is laid out in the *Timaeus*. Plato followed Empedocles in accepting earth, water, air, and fire as the four elements.[38] He envisioned a world (Universe):

> That should be a completer living being…. that it should be ageless and without disease.[39]

This was Plato's "World-Soul."[40] In contrast to the human soul, it was perfect and free from the imperfections that shackle humankind. The movement of the Universe resulted from an internal, self-moved source—the World-Soul. The same was true for the human body. The soul accounted for the body's ability to move. The human soul is also made of the same "mixture" as the World-Soul and has the same structure. In this regard, Plato saw a macrocosm-microcosm kinship between the Universe and humans, following the Pythagorean model. In support of this, Plato notes that the head, which contains the rational, intelligent force within us, is spherical like the Universe. In this way, the body mimics the heavens. The soul is the divine part of us; divine as are the stars above.[41] There was a connectedness between the two and this was the primary basis for the astronomy-medicine paradigm that was to influence physicians and astrologers through subsequent centuries. The Universe possessed "intelligence and reason"—for Plato it was a divine being. The World-Soul provides the Universe with "a divine source of unending and rational life for all time."[42]

This soul is "endowed with reason and harmony."[43] The concept of harmony is another Pythagorean theme that is to recur throughout the ages. Like Pythagoras, Plato believed the harmony of the Universe implied music. He developed a mathematical scheme of squares and cubes which he related to the musical scale.[44] Two squared was seen as a two-dimensional object; three cubed as a three-dimensional one. This echoes the Pythagorean numerical elements that were said to be the basic material of which the sublunary world was made. The timing of planetary orbital ratios had a mathematical and, thus, musical meaning for Plato.[45] He was influenced in this by Pythagoras' discovery that musical notes were related to one another in terms of mathematical ratios—2:1 for adjacent octaves; a fifth interval, 3:2 and so on.[46] Like Pythagoras, he saw harmony and music in the Universe and in humankind, thus continuing this harmonic medical theme.

Not only did Plato see the Universe as divine, but he also pictured the "fixed stars (as) living beings, divine and eternal."[47] He calls both the stars and planets "gods." These gods are the makers of humankind that "weave mortal and immortal (body and soul) together and create living creatures—bringing them to birth, giving them food, aiding growth and when they perish receive them again." [48] Plato assigns one star to care for each human soul, presaging the Christian concept of a "Guardian Angel" for each of us.[49] They are to "control and guide the mortal creature for the best, except, that is, insofar as it became a cause of evil to itself." [50] The Neo-Platonists expanded on this concept in later centuries.

There are several connections between the heavens and creatures of Earth that Plato elucidates. Suffice it to say, that these many associations gave astronomers and physicians ample support for the heaven and health linkage that is so pervasive in both the ancient world and the Middle Ages. This allows Aristotle, as we shall see next, to make the atmosphere, as Hippocrates does, a major force in human health.

Two footnotes to the Plato story are worth mentioning here. Alcmaeon was one of the first to claim divinity for the Sun, Moon, stars, and planets.[51] Also, Eudoxus, a pupil of Plato, was the first to postulate celestial spheres to explain the motions of the heavens.[52] Both of these men were physicians.

Aristotle

Aristotle (384-322 B.C.E.) was not a physician but the son of one and his writings are replete with medical references. He developed to its fullest the theoretical construct that was to be the basis for all of medicine up to the modern period. He drew heavily on the thinkers that preceded him, but was able to define this system so well that it gave a rational structure to the medical paradigm of Galen and later physicians. Galen's approach to medicine went largely unquestioned during the following centuries and Aristotle's ideas provided the warrant for Galen's medicine.

Figure 2.1
Qualities and Elements

Cold + dry = earth

Cold + moist = water

Hot + moist = air

Hot + dry = fire

The concept of opposites was pre-Socratic in origin, as noted above.[53] Aristotle, however, developed these opposites more fully and strengthened the role of the earlier pairings of "hot-cold" and "wet-dry" that ultimately formed the basis for the Galenic therapeutic system. Aristotle in his *Physics*[54] states:

> Everything that comes into being comes from its opposite or from some Intermediate between the two extremes, and everything which ceases to be turns into its opposites or into some intermediate between the two extremes.

The Intermediates are no problem for Aristotle because "the Intermediates, too, are formed from the opposites." This "non-problem" would seem to introduce a contradiction into his system since Intermediates would breed Intermediates *ad infinitum*. Aristotle, however, denies the concept of infinites making his endless Intermediates untenable.[55] This aside, the idea of opposites is essential to an understanding of medieval medicine.

Using the elements of earth, water, air, and fire and the qualities of hot, cold, wet, and dry, Aristotle refines his system of opposites as listed above:[56]

These powers, or qualities, of hot-cold, dry-moist are for Aristotle creative forces responsible for the whole of sublunary space including the human being. As such, they are the cause of health and disease. An excess or deficiency of one or more of these powers accounts for disease and reestablishing the balance of the powers restores health. From Galen's time on, all medicines, which were mostly herbs, had varying degrees of hotness, coldness, wetness, or dryness and, thus, were thought to counteract the imbalance present in a specific disease. These powers were in time to be paired with the four humors.

Having structured this system, Aristotle applies it most fully in his *Meteorology*. He combines stellar divinity with the macrocosm-microcosm pairing and, along with the principle of the opposites, is able to state:

> The world (the Earth) necessarily has certain continuity with the upper motion; consequently, all its (the Earth's) power is derived from them (the divine stars). So we must treat fire and earth and the elements like them as the material cause of the events in this world but (we) must assign causality in the sense of the originating principle of motion to the power of the eternally moving (stellar) bodies.[57]

Aristotle is saying that the four elements are the "receptacles" for the form that gives reality to all bodies. He is referring to the four causes defined in his *Metaphysics*: formal, material, efficient and final.[58] For a body to be a body it must have both matter and form and the form is provided by the stars and any power that earthly bodies possess must come from the heavens. Health or disease, which reside in earthly bodies, is a consequence of these heavenly powers and thus the stars can influence our medical well-being.

It is in the *Meteorology* that Aristotle introduces the concept of "ether," the fifth element or quintessence (literally fifth substance). Since the stars are divine, eternal, and unchanging (in contrast to the four elements), they must be composed of some divine element. All heavenly bodies, from the Moon outward, are made up of ether. This includes the Sun, Moon, planets, comets, and stars. The word "ether" is derived from αει and θειν i.e., "always to run" or "always in motion" but these roots also contain an allusion to θεοζ or god. The gods provide the eternal motion of the Universe.

Aristotle then moves to specific examples of what he means. The Sun, for example, warms the Earth by its motion, which heats the air surrounding it and thus accounts for the hot and dry qualities we sense.[59] Aristotle thought that the light of the stars and Sun came from the friction created as these bodies moved through space. Similarly, the Moon, which is wet and cold, causes dew to form on grass at night. The Moon is considered by the Ancients to be feminine and so women are primarily wet and cold. The menstrual cycle is the same length as the lunar cycle, further supporting this relationship. The light of the stars, meteors, auroras, Milky Way and comets were all thought to come from this celestial friction. They contained no fire, for the element fire was restricted to the sublunary world. Comets were considered to "foreshadow wind and drought," both of which may impact health. This cometary effect on earthly happenings is not magical; it is simply a physical effect of the comet's motion and the resulting change in the upper atmosphere. These heavenly actions accounted for heat, evaporation, condensation and "exhalation," all of which have a role to play in the workings of the world in which we live. Exhalation was the transformation of earth into water or water into air and air into fire. The four elements were considered by Aristotle to be the same changing from one to the other continually.[60] He did recognize that evaporation of bodies of water yielded rain through subsequent condensation. It was thought that healthy, drinkable water is provided by the agency of the Sun's heat what Aristotle calls the "finest and sweetest water."[61] He maintains that generation and destruction of all life on Earth is caused by the dry warmth provided by the Sun.[62] Even the "spontaneous" appearance of life (such as maggots) from putrid material is, according to Aristotle, related to solar action.[63]

The winds and clouds are also consequences of the Sun's warmth. Aristotle, following Hippocrates, attributes a variety of diseases to the several winds, depending on their direction. The rising and setting of Orion was seen as a cause of "treacherous, stormy" and, thus, unhealthy winds, especially at sea. The winds can be dry or wet, depending on their direction, which in turn relates to solar effects. He compares the winds to the hotness or coldness, wetness or dryness of the bowels, which affect digestion, all as a consequence of the Sun. How this is mediated is not clearly articulated by Aristotle.[64] Nonetheless, if there is the proper amount of heat in the bowels, food is correctly "concocted"[65] and the body remains healthy—another way the heavens impact bodily functions.

Aristotle, like most of the early Greeks, was a speculative and not an observational astronomer, though he did write extensively on astronomy in both his *Metaphysics* and *De Coelo*. The relative sections from these works will not be detailed here. They do, however, support the view that Aristotle provided a sound, logical and rational basis for the Galenic medicine that was to prove so influential in late antiquity and the Middle Ages.

The Romans

Both astronomy/astrology and medicine were active interests of the Romans.[66] Much of what passed for these two sciences, however, was drawn from the Greek thinkers who preceded them. There were, nonetheless, some significant advances made in medicine by Galen and in astronomy by Ptolemy. But before discussing the important writers of the Roman period, we must spend some time investigating the concepts of *Astronomia* and *Astrologia*.

Astronomy and Astrology

Astrology/astronomy is thought to have begun in Mesopotamia and much of the work done there was valid observational astronomy.[67] Hipparchus (second century B.C.E.) used these observations extensively in his catalog of stars and prediction of eclipses.[68] Early Egyptian horoscopes have been uncovered, though this pseudo-science was not fully developed until the Greeks refined astrology in the fourth and third centuries B.C.E. The first Mesopotamian horoscope dates to 410 B.C.E. and the Greeks followed shortly after this with their horoscopes.[69]

As with the four humors and the effect they have on personality (cholric, phlegmatic, sanguine and melancholic), similar characterizations were developed relating to the stars and other heavenly bodies. The Romans attributed the personalities of the gods to those of humans. For example, they spoke of a "jovial", "saturnine" (gloomy) or "mercurial" (eloquent) person—after planets identified with the gods Jupiter, Saturn and Mercury. These associations were strongly influenced by Greek astrology. Roman astronomy/astrology was exclusively derived from Hellenistic sources [70] but its strong influence in the Middle Ages may be attributed to the wide support given this discipline by the Roman elite.

It is not the intent of this book to deal in any detail with the pseudo-science of astrology as it is commonly represented in horoscopes. It is important for our present purposes to understand some elements of astrology as they relate to health in the ancient and medieval worlds. In the Middle Ages, the terms *Astrologia* and *Astronomia* were not clearly distinguished. McClusky[71] describes four "astronomies." These include: (1) the ancient determinations of the rising and setting of the Sun and stars related to religious rituals (2) the Easter *Computus* used in setting the date for Easter each year (3) monastic timekeeping useful in establishing times for canonical hours of prayer (4) the placement of stars and planets. The Egyptians, as we saw earlier, used ritual astronomy extensively. The ancient Greeks, starting with Thales, often practiced a "scientific" astronomy.[72] Plato, in the *Georgias*, claims that Socrates defined astronomy as, "the discipline devoted to investigating the movements of the fixed stars, the Sun, Moon and their spatial relationship to each other."[73] The last three "astronomies" defined by McClusky were primarily medieval inventions and all four would fit under the rubric of "astronomy" as we define it today. However, from the time of the Ancients up to the works of Aristarchus and Hipparchus, there was no clear distinction between astronomy and astrology. Even with Ptolemy, as we shall see later, the differentiation was not always clear and this blurred border persisted through the Middle Ages and Renaissance.

In this regard, it is helpful to divide astrology into "natural" and "judicial." [74] Natural astrology would include apparent or real relationships between the heavens and the Earth. Much of what Hippocrates and Aristotle saw as heaven and earth, cause and effect would qualify as "natural" astrology. This includes the seeming effects of the planets on earthly happenings, as well as, the meteorological changes that appear to be associated with certain maladies such as plagues, just as the Moon was thought to cause dew and regulate menstrual cycles. Judicial astrology, on the other hand, relates to horoscopes and their predictive value. [75] Natal horoscopes were (and still are by modern day astrologers) thought to foretell the personality, life events, diseases and ultimate death of a newly born baby, based solely on the exact time of his or her birth (or better yet, conception). In Rome, this was of major interest to every parent. A favorite, though illegal, pastime was to secretly cast the horoscope of the emperor. Politics were closely linked to judicial astrology at the time. [76] Out of necessity, this chapter will deal with judicial astrology only as it forms some basis for medieval medicine with emphasis primarily on natural astrology.

As we have seen, Aristotle contributed to the philosophical development of astrology and made it more psychologically palatable. [77] He viewed the Earth as the center of the Universe and the stars and planets as impacting the mundane affairs of earthly life. In a real sense, Aristotle laid the groundwork for both natural and judicial astrology. Astrology is known to have influenced many of the great men of Antiquity, including Alexander the Great and Seleucus who succeeded him. Julius Caesar, though not a strong proponent of astrology, used it for political purposes and, in fact, wrote a small treatise on stars, *De Astris*. Such notable figures as Hipparchus, Ptolemy, and Galen were all convinced, to varying degrees, of the earthly influences of the stars. [78] It was easy for these thinkers to extend the effects that the Sun had on the temperature of the air, and its impact on health, to the effects the stars and planets appeared to have on all aspects of life. They easily slid down the slippery slope from natural to judicial astrology.

As an offshoot of the Pythagorean school, numerology played a role in medicine as well. Using various calculations, a patient's prognosis could be derived from the day he or she first became sick. Numerology was often used, like judicial astrology, for a variety of personal prophecies.

Initially, astrological forecasts were used for political purposes but by the third century B.C.E., individual horoscopes came into use and, along with them, medical prognostications. These astrological "advances" soon affected all aspects of Roman life, though not all the citizens accepted astrology as a valid discipline. About 300 B.C.E., a plague spread through Rome, which prompted the government to establish the first sanctuary of Asclepius.[79] Eventually, Asclepius became the patron of iatromathematics, a system of medicine that applied astrological theories to medical practice. This system persisted through the Middle Ages and Renaissance. Various parts of the body, internal organs and diseases were placed under the influence of specific stars and constellations. As part of this "science," the concept of "critical days" developed. These critical days had to be taken into account in the treatment of individual patients, their diseases and preparation of herbal remedies.

Astrological botany dealt with herbal treatments. Certain herbs were thought to "represent" and "contain" the power of individual planets. Such drugs were expected to give the patient a direct astral benefit necessary to cure an afflicting disease. It was like reaching into the healing heavens and gathering up the planetary powers necessary to cure the patient by prescribing an herb that possessed specific stellar powers. After all, the herbs were seen as having been generated and nurtured by the stars; thus they were believed to contain the powers of stars. The harmony of the Universe, as found in astral herbs, was used to restore the harmony of a diseased mind or body.

Roman astrology was increasingly popular through the reign of Augustus Caesar (27 B.C.E-14 C.E). After Julius Caesar was assassinated, a comet appeared in the sky for seven days.[80] Augustus saw this as an indication that Julius had ascended into the heavens as a divine being. Both Nero (reigned 54-68 C.E.) and Hadrian (reigned 117-138 C.E.) were believers in the power of astrology but by the second century C.E. (c. 66-c. 176) there were imperial edicts outlawing astrology.[81] Later astrology was officially denounced by the medieval Church, though it has never gone out of vogue—witness the horoscope in every daily newspaper.

Lucretius

Lucretius (c. 96-55 B.C.E.) was a Roman poet who, "found...wonder and joy in the perceptible Universe and...workings of natural law."[82] His most notable work was *On the Nature of the Universe*. In it he deals with both astronomy and medicine. As far as we can tell he was the first to suggest the possibility of extraterrestrial life.[83] Lucretius proclaims:

> Granted, then, that empty space extends without limit in every direction and that seeds innumerable in number are rushing on countless courses through an unfathomable universe under the impulse of perpetual motion, it is in the highest degree unlikely that the earth and sky is the only one to have been created and that all those particles outside are accomplishing nothing…. You are bound therefore to acknowledge in other regions there are other earths and various tribes of men and breeds of beasts. [84]

Lucretius, in this prophetic statement, foreshadows the twentieth-century beginnings of aerospace biology and the search for extraterrestrial life.

Lucretius followed Hippocrates and Aristotle in assigning stellar influences to earthly affairs. He was, like Democritus, an atomist, and believed the Universe was made up of indivisible atoms with the "void" (vacuum) in between these particles. Using this system, he explained epidemics as follows:

> I will now explain the nature of epidemics and the sources from which the accumulated power of pestilence is able to spring a sudden devastating plague upon the tribes of men and beasts. I, in the first place, have shown above that there are certain atoms of many substances that are vital to us, and that on the other hand there must be countless others flying about that are pestiferous and poisonous. When these by some chance, have accumulated and upset the balance of the atmosphere, the air grows pestiferous. This crop of pestilence and plague either comes in through the sky from outside, like clouds or mists or very often springs from the earth itself when it has been rotted by drenching with unseasonable rains and pelting with sunbeams.[85]

This passage supports the celestial causation of disease. Lucretius also notes the effect of winds and climate on health. For example, he connects elephantiasis (a parasitic infection of the lymph glands) to the climate in Egypt, gout to the ambience in Attica and the same cause to eye problems in Achaia. "This is brought about by variations in the air that emanates from the heavens."[86] What he proposes differs little from Hippocrates and Aristotle. We have already seen they believed solar heat was responsible for both generation and destruction of life. Lucretius also injects the idea of atmospheric disharmony or disorder as a cause of disease. His atomism allows him additional rational support for both diseases from the heavens, as well as the possibility of extraterrestrial life, so that he adds a few new twists to the theoretical basis for medical practice in contemporary Rome.

Cicero

Cicero (106-43 B.C.E.) is the most famous of Roman orators. In his *On Divination*, he specifically argues against the practice of predicting the future, whether by astrology, augury or other forms of divination.[87] He associates the beginnings of astrology with the "Assyrians" who observed the heavens and "began to take notice of …the paths and motions of the stars…(and who) handed down to their posterity information as to what was indicated by their various positions and revolutions."[88] Cicero claims that many Pythagoreans, Stoics and Peripatetics (Aristotelians) supported divination in its various forms. Cicero dismisses such beliefs as mere superstition. We should "laugh at soothsayers" and "despise…Babylonian astrologers."[89] In so doing, he rejects judicial astrology. However, he admits of two types of divination: "one partaking of art and the other wholly devoid of it."[90] The former he refers to as "natural divination"—similar to natural astrology. The human soul is influenced by the divine soul i.e. from heavenly divinities (stars and planets) but through reason and the "contemplation of nature," one can "anticipate things to come."[91] Those partaking of art "have learned to judge of what is told by observation." These men (and women), he goes on, proceed by way of "reason." Here Cicero seems to indicate, that by experiencing past events and making reasoned judgments based on these observations, one can predict future happenings. However, those who do not make measured predictions based on "observation" of "particular signs" but rather respond to some "excitement of mind" are charlatans. This might be compared to the modern day weatherman who, after many observations, and aided by the computer, can "predict" future weather. Having said this, Cicero goes on to accept prognostications made via dream interpretation, auguries, auspices, prophecies and oracles, especially the Oracle at Delphi, as long as they are facilitated by the "gods." "All that happens to men may happen by the direction of heaven." [92] As proof of this, he cites many predictions reported over the centuries that have proven to be true and accurate. He quotes past "authorities" including Thales,[93] Solon, Plato, and Aristotle, to support his views. He also notes that physicians and ships pilots can predict future events. He includes the "intonation of voice" as part of predicting the future, thus including music (harmony) in the process of divination. Predictions "from the stars are founded on the accurate observations of many centuries." He goes on to say:

> Now it is certain that a long course of careful observation, carefully conducted for a series of ages, usually brings with it an incredible accuracy of knowledge; and this can exist even without the inspiration of the gods, when it has once been ascertained by constant observation what follows after each omen and what is indicated by each prodigy.[94]

Cicero is not talking about astronomical observation of the type Hipparchus accomplished, but rather, effects he attributes to various celestial events, such as comets, which, according to Cicero and other "authori-ties," are often followed by certain catastrophes. The majority of such predictions he ascribes to the:

> Nature of the gods, from which, as the wisest men acknowledge, we derive and enjoy the energies of our souls, and as everything is filled and pervaded by divine intelligence and eternal sense, it follows of necessity that the soul of man must be influenced by its kindred with the soul of the Deity.[95]

He goes on to develop a "soul out-of-body" experience to explain the divinely induced predictions arising from dreams, trances, oracles, auguries etc. In effect, what Cicero does is to support, if not judicial, at least natural astrology, thus, continuing the trend stemming from the Greeks and, in turn, allowing Galen and others to strengthen the astronomical underpinnings of ancient and medieval medicine. Cicero does not necessarily claim that the heavenly signs are the causes of such misfortunes but rather are harbingers of things to come. He also did not affirm the inevitability of predicted events; they could, at times be altered.

In addition, he describes the use of herbs and roots by "physicians as good for the bites of beasts, for complaints of the eyes, and for wounds, the power and nature of which reason has never been explained...yet both the art and inventor of these medicines have gained universal approval from their utility." [96] He accepts the usefulness of *scammony* as a purga-tive and *aristolochia* in the treatment of serpent bites—the latter having been discovered in a dream. This affirmation of herbal medicines also was supportive of therapies used later in the Middle Ages. He as well, espouses the idea of Fortuna, the goddess of fate, a concept which is to play a role in future medicine, as well.[97]

Cicero's approach to divination is paradoxical, in that he begins by denigrating the concept wholesale. Using ancient authority and "ob-servation," he rescues divination with only a few exceptions, which he labels divination without "art." His reliance on authority is a common thread throughout ancient and medieval thought, not to be questioned until the thirteenth century and more robustly in the sixteenth century. His concept of observation is much the same as that of Hippocrates and Aristotle. They all failed in not distinguishing between anecdotal and scientific observation. Not until statistical methods emerged during the Enlightenment, was true science to surface.[98] In essence, Cicero furthered the heaven and health relationship, giving a passing nod, along the way, to harmony in health.

Manilius

Marcus Manilius (first century C.E.) wrote the *Astronomica* around 14-27 C.E.[99] This work was the last of the great Roman epic poems and deals with astronomy and astrology. Manilius was a true judicial astrologer and in his writings develops a fairly complete astrological system with all its natal horoscopic predictions of future life events. He discusses cosmology,[100] including the four elements,[101] discord and harmony in the Universe.[102] Harmony is a recurrent theme in the *Astronomica*.[103] His writings contain aspects of the Stoic cosmogony and cosmology. He sees all celestial bodies, including the Earth, as spherical and suspended in space.[104] He also discusses lunar eclipses and climatic zones. The constellations are described with emphasis on the signs of the zodiac. He notes the stick figures represented by the constellations and explains their "stingy" forms as the Divinity's unwillingness to burden the heavens with too much fire. Manilius affirms the immutability of the stars, as first postulated by Plato. Many of his descriptions of the constellations are likely taken from Aratus' *Phenomona*,[105] whose work was often referred to in Antiquity and the Middle Ages. He does not identify Ophiuchus with Asclepius, as others have done.[106] Mention is made of the Arctic and Antarctic circles,[107] the summer and winter tropics, the ecliptic[108] and the tilt of the Earth's axis.[109] He includes the Milky Way in his "fixed Circles" and discusses the various theories of the Milky Way proposed by the Ancients, including Democritus' idea that the Milky Way is composed of many small stars[110]—a concept that did not take hold until Galileo's time.[111] He covers comets, advancing three theories for their cause including inflammatory earth vapors ignited by dry air, stars attracted to and then released by the Sun and finally God's means of warning humankind of impending calamities.[112]

Figure 2.2
Zodiac Anatomy

Aries: head	Libra: loins
Taurus: neck	Scorpio: groin
Gemini: arms	Sagittarius: thighs
Cancer: breast	Capricorn: knees
Leo: sides	Aquarius: shanks
Virgo: belly	Pisces: feet

Manilius deals with a great number of strictly astronomical concepts, nonetheless, the *Astronomina's* focus is mainly on astrological beliefs. For example, he assigns the anatomical parts of the body to the several signs of the zodiac.[113]. These associations, as we have already seen, were to play an important role in medieval medicine. He is convinced that the heavens determine all events on Earth, including the course of human lives from birth to death. He speaks of "the secrets of the skies by which all things are ruled"[114] Further, he writes:

> All things moved to the will and disposition of heaven, as the constellations by their varied array assign different destinies.[115]

This is a theme repeated many times by Manilius. Like Hippocrates, he relates body habitus to geography:

> The land of Egypt, flooded by the Nile, darkens the body more mildly owing to the inundation of its fields; it is a country nearer to us and its climate imparts a medium tone.[116]
> Germany, towering high with tall offspring, is blond;
> Gaul is tinged to a less degree with a near-related redness.[117]

In this passage, these features are ascribed to the different signs of the zodiac that "lay claim to different lands" as much as to geography.

He goes on to give the geometry of the horoscope with its many relationships, which will not be outlined here and can be found in any textbook of astrology.[118] Horoscope predictions are "based on the belief that the zodiac and planets, as they ceaselessly revolve around the Earth exert different influences according to their different positions relative to the native" (new born child.)[119] Certain parts of the horoscope wheel were thought to have power over various areas of ones life including health. He counts twelve "athla" or "houses" (similar to the hours of the day on the face of a clock). The eleventh "athla" deals with health. The seventh athla controls "dangers" including violent death. The length of life can be forecast from the horoscope as well. And in true Stoic fashion, Fortuna or Fate plays a major role in ones health and happiness.

A few examples of health related aspects of Manilius' *Astronomica* will be covered in order to give a sense of his system and how it influenced later medicine. In speaking of Sirius, the Dog Star, he says:

> …No star comes on mankind more violently or causes more trouble when it departs. Now it rises shivering with cold, now it leaves a radiant world open to the heat of the Sun. Thus, it moves the world to either extreme and brings opposite effects. Those who…observe it ascending when it returns at its first rising learn of the various outcomes of harvests and seasons, what state of health lies in store and what measure of harmony.[120]

This description of the effects of Sirius is an example of natural astrology, though the causes and effects cited are spurious. Most of his *Astronomica* deals with judicial aspects of this "noble science" (astrology).[121] But the quotation above contains some of the flavor we taste in Hippocrates and Aristotle. Both types of astrology, as we shall see, have their effects on medieval medicine. Much of what he has to say deals with natal horoscopes and the future they portend[122] or with mythical allusions. An example of the latter is found in his view of the Milky Way, which he describes as a "river of milk" that nourishes the young Jupiter, though in the same paragraph, he mentions Democritus' view of the Galaxy as a "host of stars." This insight, if Manilius believed it, was precocious, indeed, for the truth of this statement was not to be proven until the telescope came along. Manilius relates the appearance of comets to the occurrence of plagues and describes in some detail Theucydites' Plague, which ravished Athens in 430 B.C.E. taking even the life of its great leader, Pericles.[123]

> Death comes with these celestial torches (comets) that threaten Earth with the blaze of (funeral) pyres unceasing, since heaven and nature's self are stricken and seem doomed to share men's tomb.

With these ominous words of Manilius, we move on to the great Stoic philosopher Seneca, whose life scenario is no more encouraging. Manilius wrote the *Astronomia* during the height of Roman interest in astrology. It was a "song" that is, an epic poem that even Goethe praised (though he denounced its astrological content).[124] It contains a great deal of true astronomy, some of which was new. His cosmology accords with the Ancients before him. Events in the lives of humans are caused by divine, heavenly bodies. The organization of the Universe is based on its pervasive harmony. These two beliefs confirm the theories that sustained medicine going forward. Manilius impacted philosophers for a century after his death.[125] One of these was Seneca, the Stoic philosopher.

Seneca

Another influence that promoted the development of judicial astrology in Rome was the popularity of Stoic philosophy. Seneca (4 B.C.E. – c. 65 C.E.) was a leading Roman Stoic and adviser to Nero until he fell out of favor (possibly related to a coup against the emperor) and was forced to commit suicide.[126]

Stoicism was the most popular Roman (initially Greek) philosophical system for several centuries. Its appeal to astrologers lay in its fatalistic principles. Fortuna, the goddess of fortune, controlled all aspects of ones life and our role is to be resigned to the fate the gods have chosen for us. The Stoics saw the world as a single, great community with everyone related harmoniously under divine reason, that is, the spirit of the Universe or Nature.[127] It is a person's duty to live in conformity with the divine will. This concept fed into the determinism of astrology. Seneca, though a non-physician, was not immune to making medical pronouncements such as, "Restlessness…is symptomatic of a sick mind" and, "a wound will not heal over if it is being made the subject of experiments with different ointments." [128] Though little more will be said about Stoicism, this is not to diminish its effect on future medicine; it provided another theoretical support for astrology and, subsequently, Roman Catholic theology, so dominant up to the Reformation. As we shall see, acceptance of ones situation in life was integral to the theology of the Middle Ages. Though times were hard in this life, if one follows the laws of God and His Church, a much better life lies ahead in heaven. Heavenly healing was a religious theme of the medieval Church. The heavens and its harmony played a role in health. Stoicism, thus, provided impetus to the ideas that were to be so important in the Middle Ages.

Claudius Galenus

Claudius Galenus (c. 130-200 C.E.) was born in Asia Minor.[129] As a teenager, he may have been an attendant or "therapeute" at the temple of Asclepius and it is here in Pergamum, his native city, that he studied medicine. Early in his career, he was surgeon to the gladiators at Pergamum, which allowed him to gain some knowledge of human anatomy. His anatomy, however, was Hippocratic in focus[130] and, though he was a talented dissector,[131] all This work was on animals,[132] which led to anatomical errors that were perpetuated for centuries. At age thirty-two, he traveled to Rome. In time, he became a medical advisor to the Emperor Marcus Aurelius.

Galen followed the teachings of Hippocrates but elaborated on and classified[133] his system and it was in this "Galenic" form that medieval medicine ultimately was practiced.[134] Galen believed strongly that the best physician must be a philosopher.[135] The doctor had to be a master of the "Arts" which included logic, geometry, and astronomy among other disciplines:

> It was the opinion of Hippocrates that astronomy (and therefore the study of geometry) is of central relevance to the study of medicine.

Of course, all the subjects of the *Trivium* (logic, rhetoric and grammar) and *Quadrivium* (arithmetic, music, geometry and astronomy) were included in Galen's "Arts." The physician had to be a "philosopher", which would today include both liberal arts and the sciences.

Hippocrates, according to Galen, had separated himself from cosmological speculations, emphasizing experimental medicine instead. Galen followed these principles, but both men made room for heavenly influences in their practices. Galen's emphasis was more on prognosis[136] than diagnosis and, as with Hippocrates, he believed strongly in the healing powers of "Nature." [137] He affirms the importance of environmental factors as presented in Hippocrates'*Airs, Waters, Places,*[138] once again joining heaven and health. Galen used several of the earlier concepts that the Ancients had proposed which linked the outer "spheres" with the sublunary world. One of these was the idea of "pneuma," "spiritus," or breath.[139, 140] The pneuma had two meanings: one relating to inspired air, which was associated with the principle of "vital heat," so important in the maintenance of life; the other was tied to the vegetative and animal vital principles or "nature" of a being. This nature is connected to "Nature" in the more universal sense and is another philosophical concept uniting the macrocosm with the microcosm. A further astronomical bond is provided by Aristotle's "ether"—the stuff out of which the stars and planets are made. Galen ties the divine soul to the inner soul of humans—the human soul being separate from the four elements. The quintessence is related to the form which, when united to matter, accounts for "substance" or true being, in this case the human being. The "pneuma" and "ether" could be considered analogous concepts. These ideas persisted into the Renaissance and are seen in the writings of astrologer-physicians of that period such as Paracelsus, who will be reviewed below.[141]

As noted earlier, the Galenic system of medicine relied heavily on Hippocrates and his School. Part of Galen's medicine combined the structure of the four elements, earth, water, air, and fire, with the four powers, hot, cold, dry and wet, along with the four humors, yellow and black bile, blood and phlegm, as discussed earlier.[142] As also outlined above, these formed a unified theory of health and disease that, in fact, emanates from the cosmology of the Ancients. This system was developed most fully by Galen and formed the basis for all of medieval medicine—etiology, signs and symptoms, therapy, and prognosis.

Galen writes at length about the function of various herbs such as "safflower and the cuidian berry, which do not draw phlegm from the body, but actually make it" [143] On the other hand, certain cholagogues, (herbs that increase bile) will augment the flow of yellow bile, thus, ridding the body of its excess. A purgative that attracts a given humor will also remove an excess or "superfluity" of that humor. Other herbs may increase a bodily humor when it is deficient. Galen believed that each drug attracts that humor which is proper to it." [144] All diseases were due to either an excess or deficiency of one or more humors and therapy was aimed at removing or replacing this humoral imbalance in the afflicted patient and restoring the body's balance (harmony). As discussed before, these imbalances are caused by influences from the atmosphere, stars or planets and the herbs had the power to usurp the workings of these celestial bodies and counteract their adverse effects.

Galen believed there were seasonal effects of some therapies and ties these to the four humors:

> Is it not also the fact that in summer the yellow bile is evacuated in greater quantity by the same drugs and in winter phlegm, and that in a young man more bile is evacuated, and in an old man more phlegm?…Thus, if you give in the summer season a drug which attracts phlegm to a young man of a lean and warm habit, who has lived neither idly nor too luxuriously, you will with great difficulty evacuate a very small quantity of this humor, and you will do the man the utmost harm. On the other hand, you give him a cholagogues, you will produce an abundant evacuation and not injure him at all. [145]

Galen identifies the seasons, body habitus, and character of the patient as important considerations in the healing process. As with Hippocrates, he is aware of the therapeutic properties of proper diet and exercise.

Galen uses the magnetic qualities of loadstone to "prove," "that there are in all bodies certain faculties by which they attract their own proper qualities." [146] He also notes that chaff is attracted by amber. [147] According to Galen, it is the attractive powers of the body that herbs mimic and, in so doing allow the body to restore the balance of humors. The herb can attract nutriments necessary to form a healing humor or to act as a cathartic to draw superfluous humors from the body.

One other Galenic concept is worth mentioning in support of our thesis. Galen believed that herbs "represent" and contain the powers of individual planets." [148] In the astromathematical system, parts of the body are related to specific constellations or planets. Medical therapy is based on this relationship, that is, individual patients and herbs have a special connection with the skies. The position of celestial bodies determines the effect of a given drug on a given patient, so that certain treatments could only be administered with benefit (and not harm) on those days prescribed by the heavens. This concept played a major role in medicine of the Middle Ages, as we shall see.

It is hard to overstate Galen's impact on ancient and medieval medicine. He was a prolific writer (in Greek), producing twenty volumes of medical information. His works were held to be sacrosanct and during the Enlightenment were stubbornly followed even in the face of contrary evidence. Why this was so, is the topic of a later section.

Ptolemy

Claudius Ptolemaeus (c.100-173 c.e.) is the most noted astronomer of Antiquity and his *Almagest* was the most sophisticated astronomical treatise yet written.[149] It was to be the standard astronomical work until Copernicus' *De Revolutionibus* published in 1543.[150] Ptolemy's cosmological system, with its geocentrism, deferents epicycles and equants[151] (see Appendix) formed the basis of virtually all astronomical thought up to the Copernican Revolution.[152] In spite of his astronomical and mathematical prowess, Ptolemy was dedicated to what he called, "astronomical prognostication."[153] At the end of the *Almagest,* [154] Ptolemy devoted four books to this topic, referred to as the *Tetrabiblos*. A reading of these books leaves no doubt that he was a dedicated astrologer with an appetite for natural as well as a strong taste for judicial astrology. Ptolemy pontificates early in the *Tetrabiblos*:

> That a certain power, derived from the ethereal nature, is diffused over and pervades the whole atmosphere of the Earth, is clearly evident to all men. [155]

In other words, the ether of the divine stars (and planets) has influence throughout this world of ours. And this diffused ether is found in our bodies and mediates health and disease—echoes from Aristotle destined to reverberate through the subsequent centuries. In his *Almagest* Ptolemy,[156] in fact, performs some horoscopic calculations, but in general, the *Almagest* is free of astrological material. Ptolemy goes on to say:

> The stars likewise (as well as the planets) in performing their revolutions produce many impressions on the Ambient. They cause heat, winds, and storms to the influence of which earthly things are conformably subjected.... And further, the mutual configuration of all these heavenly bodies, by commingling the influences with which each is separately invested, produces a multiplicity of changes. The power of the Sun, however, predominates, because it is more generally distributed; the others either co-operate with the Sun's power or diminish its effect; the Moon more frequently and more plainly performs this at her conjunction.[157]

Then to solidify the genethalogical (natal) influences he says:

All bodies…are subjected to the motion of the stars, but also that the impregnation and growth of the seed from which all bodies proceed, are framed and molded by the quality existing in the Ambient at the time of such impregnation. [158]

In brief, the course of our lives is etched in stone by the configuration of the heavens at the moment of conception. Having said this, Ptolemy then takes the next step and states unequivocally that if one is knowledgeable in the movement of the stars, it is possible:

To make predictions concerning the proper quality of the seasons…(and) similar prognostications concerning the destiny and disposition of every human being. [159]

Ptolemy devotes the first two chapters of Book I of the *Tetrabiblos* to establishing astrology as a true science. He points out the accuracy of predictions made by the Ancients and how astrology has proven time and again to be a practical and predictable method of foretelling both personal and political events. It seems clear to him that the heavens permeate and control all happenings in the sublunary world of humans—both good and bad happenings.

He urges the physician, in dealing with "the sick person as well as his disease" to include not only seasons, habitus, diet, symptoms, etc. but also the "motions of the heavens," which are just as important as these other characteristics of disease. [160] He goes on to say that the physician after consulting the heavens:

Indicates (a medical event) shall absolutely take place; and…that another event shall not happen…. It is this manner that the experienced physician, accustomed to the observation of disease, foresees that some will be inevitably mortal and that others are susceptible of cure.[161]

Thus, astrology can aid the physician in prognostications regarding the course of a disease, which makes him appear knowledgeable and erudite—often not saving the patient but saving face!

Ptolemy is not entirely fatalistic in his medical prognostications. He allows for the beneficial effects of medical therapy, but such treatment must be mixed with astronomical finesse:

Without an understanding of the stars, medicines will be improperly prescribed and harm done to the patient. [162]

Ptolemy deals at some length with the four elements, qualities, temperaments and humors in a classic Galenic fashion. He attributes heat and dryness to the Sun, moisture and some heat to the Moon, cold and dryness to Saturn. Mars is dry with some heat; Jupiter has moderate heat and dryness; Venus has moderate heat and moisture; and Mercury may produce dryness or moisture, heat or cold, depending on its relationship to the Sun and its velocity. These qualities cause disease, and herbs with contrary qualities, can overcome these ill effects and restore health. Ptolemy basically follows Galen but uses a more rigid astrological structure. He also catalogues the effects of the zodiac constellations. As an example, Taurus mediates effects similar to Venus. Venus is, of course, a "feminine" sign but Taurus, paradoxically, is also considered "feminine." This is true in present day astrology as well. It is not necessary to spend time on Ptolemy's specific "presciences" or predictions and the celestial bases he uses for these predictions. In general, Ptolemy follows the astrology of the Greeks and Romans, much of which is current today. The purpose here is simply to demonstrate that Ptolemy maintains the same ancient theoretical themes that went on to influence medicine of the Middle Ages. He is simply transmitting the "wisdom" of the Ancients to future generations of healers.

Firmicus

Julius Firmicus Maternus, who lived in the fourth century C.E., wrote the *Mathesos* or *Theory of Astrology* about 334 C.E.[163] The word *Mathesos* means "learning" and Firmicus considered his *Mathesos* a truly scientific writing.[164] Such "learning" formed the basis of the Liberal Arts, first studied in ancient Greece. The medieval system of learning, as noted above, consisted of the *Trivium* (grammar, logic and rhetoric) and the *Quadrivium* (arithmetic, music, geometry and astronomy). *Mathesos* had two meanings in the Middle Ages. The one indicating true learning, as in the Liberal Arts, and the other denoting "superstition," as astrology was thought to be by many intellectuals, though this was not so for Firmicus. The Liberal Arts and their role in medieval medicine will be covered in detail later. In the late Roman and early Christian periods, Firmicus' *Mathesos*, was considered a proper treatise and, even though it lost some of its academic luster in the early Middle Ages, partially due to condemnation by the Church, this work had a major impact on institutions of higher learning.

Firmicus considered the *Mathesos* not only scientific but also "a pure and high form of philosophy." [165] He based this opinion on the Stoic concept of *"symopatheia"*, that is, the intimate relationship of all parts of the Universe, including the stars and humans—a theme we have seen before. The deterministic aspect of Stoicism, so strong in early Roman astrology, is maintained by Firmicus in the extreme. He includes snatches of Hellenistic science and stellar mythology, as well as all the well-developed astrological relationships so important to the astrologers of this period. He speaks of twelve signs of the zodiac and the seven "planets" including Mercury, Venus, Mars, Jupiter, Saturn, the Moon, plus the Sun. He uses the Babylonian system of 360° to divide the sky. Each zodiac sign covers 30° and these are further divided into "decans" of 10°, each division having its own astrological significance. The zodiac signs moved through the sky from season to season. There were also twelve "houses" that did not move and through which the zodiac signs traveled on a continuous basis. We have seen the "houses" before. Each "house" had meaning related to various aspect of life, such as, parents, children, health, death etc. And there were also "sextiles" and "trienes" that had to do with the 60° or 120° relationships (aspects) of four or three constellations or planets.[166] There were also oppositions (180° separation) and conjunctions (objects within 7° of each other) of "planets." And, if a planet were found in a constellation, that configuration had meaning as well. The most crucial of connections was the sign under which one was born (or conceived). This sign was the zodiac constellation that the Sun was in at that time. Firmicus includes ascendants (the number of degrees above the horizon that a zodiac sign was in at the time of birth) and many more such relationships.[167] A horoscope consisted of all these relationships as they are at the very instant of birth. All ones life was determined by the happenstance of the stars and planets at this "natal" time. It is a very complex system and, though it has changed little over the centuries, its interpretation has evolved to meet modern needs and tendencies in our present culture. As an example, in Firmicus" *Mathesos*, violent death is predicted by numerous heavenly configurations, whereas today violent deaths, which are less common, are rarely predicted. Much of Firmicus' *Mathesos* is based on the work of Vettius Valens who was a contemporary of Ptolemy.[168] Valens was also a Roman, though he was born in Antioch, lived in Alexandria and wrote in Greek. His major work was *Anthology* (of astrology), for which there is no English translation and according to Tester[169] is difficult to comprehend at best. At the beginning of the second book of the *Anthology*, Vettius lists the three constellations that are 120° apart, along with the four elements of Greek philosophy and medicine[170] thus continuing the medical link between the elements, humors and "powers" of hot-cold, dry-wet. As an example, the constellations of Aries, Leo, and Sagittarius are "attributed" to the Sun and, thus, are connected with the element of Fire. Diseases caused by a "superfluity" of fire (such as a fever) could be due to the presence in the sky of Aries, Leo, and Sagittarius at the time the disorder began and would respond to an herbal remedy that was cold rather than hot and wet rather than dry, that is, the opposite qualities of fire. The following gives a sense of Firmicus' prognostications:

> But if the part of Fortune is found in the tenth house, that is, on the M.C. (Medium Coeli = mid-heaven) or in the eleventh in which the M.C. is often found and if the waxing Moon is there, moving over toward Saturn or with him; and if the Sun is on the ascendant, this will make the natives fortunate, blessed, noble, with the greatest power. But it also indicates afflictions and illness.[171]

Astrologers and physicians were knowledgeable in all astronomical associations. Firmicus in the *Mathesos* covers a plethora of medical problems, giving the astrological configurations associated with each. These include madness, "burning and painful fevers", early death, kypho-scoliosis (hunchback), violent death, drowning, being burned alive, blindness, accidents, demonic possession, infertility, pestilence, long life, amputations, death at birth, anxiety, gluttony, suicide and many more, all given with the celestial sign causing these disorders.[172] This complex system of stellar relationships took a long time to master.

The statement is often made that astrology contributed significantly to the understanding of astronomy. It is likely this is not true. Neugebauer and von Hoesen[173] note that in the *Anthology* and elsewhere, the mathematics used for the time of rising of the Sun, for example, is rudimentary and more sophisticated methods had been developed by the time of Vettius, but were not incorporated into his calculations. These authors believe that astrology was more a "tag along" than a leader in the growth of astronomy. Another point to be made in this regard is that neither the Greeks nor Romans were stargazers. Even Ptolemy, in writing the *Almagest*, is thought to have relied heavily on Hipparchus and the Babylonians, though undoubtedly he did gather data from personal observations of the heavens as well.[174]

Thus, the Ancients laid a rational, if fallacious, foundation for their medicine and the subsequent medical practice of the Middle Ages. Astrology played an important role in this process but it was not always fully accepted throughout a given culture and natural astrology was a more persistent feature of later medicine. Astrology actually began to wane during the early Middle Ages, only to resurface in the Renaissance as the Enlightenment was beginning. For a time there was an anachronistic coexistence of the astrologer-physician, such as the Elizabethan physicians, Robert Fludd alongside such medical masters as William Harvey.[175]

Fludd, a confirmed astrologer, was the first to support Harvey's [176] ideas concerning circulation. More will be said of this later.

As we have seen, the heavens were intimately linked to the Earth and its inhabitants. The stars were divine, composed of ether and in sympathy with the sublunary world. The fifth element, ether, along with the four unstable and changeable elements made up the Universe. The atmosphere was similarly impacted by the heavens and in turn affected all of us on Earth in both health and sickness. We are the microcosms and, as such, intimately tied to the macrocosm. We are inextricably united to the macrocosm and what happens to us, health-wise and otherwise, is bound to the macrocosm as a whole. If we are in harmony with the heavens health follows; if disharmonious with the celestial realm, disease ensues. And, depending on the system a physician espouses, so too, depends his medical theory and practice. Let us see how the medicine of the Middle Ages plays out.

Notes

1.   Neugebauer, O. 1969. *The Exact Sciences in Antiquity* (New York: Dover).
2.   Casson, L. 2001. *Everyday Life in Ancient Egypt* (Baltimore, MD: Johns Hopkins University Press), p. 60.
3.   Ibid., p. 61.
4.   Bauval, R. and Gilbert, A. 1994. *The Orion Mystery* (New York: Three Rivers Press).
5.   Johnson, P. 1999. *The Civilization of Ancient Egypt* (New York: HarperCollins).
6.   Bauval, R. and Gilbert, A., 1994 *Orion Mystery*, p. 24.
7.   Edwards, I. E. S. 1993. *The Pyramids of Egypt* (New York: Penguin), p. 34.
8.   Johnson, P. 1999. *The Civilization of Ancient Egypt* (New York: HarperCollins), p. 22.
9.   Guthrie, K. S. 1987. *The Pythagorean Source Book and Library* (Grand Rapids, MI: Phanes Press).
10.   Ibid., p. 139.
11.   Aristotle. 1952. *Aristotle's Metaphysics*, i 5 986 a 22, trans. R. Hope (Ann Arbor: University of Michigan Press).
12.   Aristotle. 1952. *Aristotle's Metaphysics*, 986a, (New York, NY: Columbia University Press) p. 15.
13.   Numbers as metaphysical entities appear not to have been fully comprehended by the Ancients, including Aristotle, who did not accept Pythagoras' metaphysical system.
14.   Guthrie, K. S. 1987. *Pythagorian Source Book*, p. 61.
15.   Ibid., Iamblichus, p. 61.
16.   Ibid., Porphyry, p. 126.
17.   Ibid., p. 127.
18.   Ibid., Porphyry, p. 130.
19.   Ibid., Porphyry, p. 134.
20.   Ibid., Photus, p. 139.
21.   Hippocrates 1923, *Writings*, vol. I-IV, Loeb Classics, trans. W. H. S. Jones (London: Harvard University Press), p. xi.

22.   Ibid., p. 16. Aristotle is uncertain as to who first developed the concept of opposites—Pythagoras or Alcmaeon.
23.   Ibid.
24.   Lambridis, H. 1976. *Empedocles* (University AL: University of Alabama Press) p. 20.
25.   Ibid., p 30.
26.   Hippocrates. 1923. *Writings*, p. xiv.
27.   Ibid., vol. II, pp. 63-125.
28.   Hippocrates. 1923. *Writings*, vol. I, p 73.
29.   Guthrie, K. S. 1987, *Pythagorian Source Book*, pp. 103-105.
30.   Hippocrates. 1923. *Writings*, vol. I, p. 99.
31.   Ibid., p. xlvii.
32.   Ibid., *Ancient Medicine*, p. 41.
33.   Ibid., p. xlviii.
34.   Ibid.
35.   Ibid.
36.   Ibid., p. x.vi.
37.   Plato. 1978. *The Republic of Plato*, trans. F. M. Cornford (New York: Oxford University Press), pp. xxvii, 217-218.
38.   Plato. 1977. *Timaeus and Critias* (London: Penguin Books), p. 44.
39.   Ibid., p. 45.
40.   Ibid., pp. 46-47.
41.   Ibid., p. 61.
42.   Ibid., p. 50.
43.   Ibid.
44.   Ibid., p. 48.
45.   It takes Mercury eighty-eight days to make one orbit around the Sun; Venus, 225 days: Mars, 687 days; Jupiter, twelve years and Saturn, thirty years. These ratios are roughly 2.5 (Mercury to Venus) 3, (Venus to Mars) 6 (Mars to Jupiter) and 16 (Jupiter to Saturn). These were considered to demonstrate the same kind of harmony found in the musical scale. Kepler made much of these ratios in the seventeenth century. See his *Harmonies of the World*.
46.   Plato. 1978. *Republic*, p. 249.
47.   Plato. 1977. *Timaeus and Critias*, p. 50.
48.   Ibid., p. 57.
49.   Ibid., p. 58.
50.   Ibid., p. 59.
51.   Aristotle. 1984. "De Anima," 405a 29, *The Complete Works of Aristotle* (Princeton, NJ: Princeton University Press) p. 646.
52.   Crowe, M. J. 1990. *Theories of the World from Antiquity to the Copernican Revolution* (New York: Dover), pp. 23-25.
53.   Sambursky, S. 1956. *The Physical World of the Greeks*, trans. M. Dagut (Princeton, NJ: Princeton University Press) p. 91.
54.   Aristotle. 1999. *Physics*, 188b21 (New York: Oxford University Press), p. 21.
55.   Hot + cold = warm; warm + cold = lukewarm; lukewarm + cold = tepid, *ad infinitum.*
56.   Sambursky, S. 1956. *Physical World*, p. 91.
57.   Op. cit. Aristotle 1984, pp. 55-56.
58.   Op. cit. Aristotle, 1952, Book alpha, 7. Formal cause is the "form" that is added to matter to make any individual or physical thing be what it is to be. Form is not otherwise defined. Material cause is prime matter, which allows form to be

expressed in a physical way. Efficient cause is the force or power that makes a thing come into existence by combining form with prime matter. Final cause is the purpose or end for which a thing is intended. Formal and material causes are strictly metaphysical concepts and cannot be conceptualized in one's imagination. Prime matter, for example, has no physical existence until united with form. Aristotle uses the analogy of a bronze statue. The shape of the statue is the form, bronze is the material cause, the artist is the efficient cause and the final cause is its aesthetic value. The analogy falls short of really explaining his four causes.

59.   Aristotle. 1984. *Meteorology,* 341a19-21. p. 558.
60.   Aristotle. 1984. *On Generation and Corruption,* 334a24-25, p. 547.
61.   Aristotle 1984, *Meteorology,* 354b26, p.577.
62.   Aristotle. 1942. *Generation of Animals,* 777b30, Loeb Classics, trans. A. L. Peck (London: Harvard University Press) p. 481.
63.   Aristotle. 1984. *History of Animals,* 547b18, *"Generation of Animals,"* 778a4, *The Complete Works of Aristotle* (Princeton, NJ: Princeton University Press), pp. 864, 1203.
64.   Aristotle 1984, *Meteorology,* 361a5, p. 585.
65.   Concoction comes from the Greek "to boil." In Galenic medicine, it has a more specific meaning. Food was concocted in the bowels and thus made healthy and utilizable by the body. This process was more than simply heating ingested food, though it was believed that digestion was largely a matter of heating food. Food was transformed by concoction into a form that allowed blood to be made in the liver from foodstuffs.
66.   Cramer, F. H. 1954. *Astrology in Roman Law and Politics* (Philadelphia, PA: American Philosophical Society).
67.   Neugebauer, O. and van Hoesen, H. B. 1959. *Exact Sciences.*
68.   Ruggles, C. and Hoskin, M. 1999. *The Cambridge Concise History of Astronomy,* ed. M. Hoskin (Cambridge: Cambridge University Press), p. 31.
69.   Cramer, F. H. 1954. *Astrology,* p. 3.
70.   Ibid., p. 4.
71.   McCluskey, S.C. 1998, *Astronomers and Cultures in Early Medieval Europe* (New York: Cambridge University Press), pp. x-xi.
72.   Cramer, F. H. 1954. *Astrology,* p. 3.
73.   Ibid.
74.   Tester, S. J. 1999. *Western Astrology,* p. 178.
75.   Orion, R. 1999. *Astrology for Dummies* (New York: IDG Books Worldwide).
76.   Cramer, F. H. 1954. *Astrology.*
77.   Ibid., p. 9.
78.   Ibid., p. 18.
79.   Ibid., p. 45.
80.   Ibid., p. 78.
81.   Ibid., p. 241.
82.   Lucretius. 1986. *On the Nature of the Universe,* trans. R. E. Latham (New York: Penguin Books), p. 10.
83.   Koerner, D. and Levay, S. 2000. *Here Be Dragons: The Scientific Quest for Extraterrestrial Life* (New York: Oxford University Press), p. 4.
84.   Lucretius. 1986. *On the Nature of the Universe,* p. 91.
85.   Ibid., p. 250.
86.   Ibid., p. 251.
87.   Cicero, M. T. 1997. *On Divination,* trans. C. D. Yonge (Amherst, NY: Prometheus Books).

88. Ibid., p. 141.
89. Ibid., p. 161.
90. Ibid., p. 159.
91. Ibid., p. 190.
92. Ibid., p. 193.
93. Ibid. Thales is said to have been the first to predict a solar eclipse.
94. Ibid., p. 189.
95. Ibid., p. 190.
96. Ibid., p. 146.
97. Ibid., p. 196.
98. Struik, D. J. 1948. *A Concise History of Mathematics* (New York: Dover).
99. Manilius. 1927. *Astronomica*, Loeb Classics, trans. G. P. Goold (London: Harvard University Press).
100. Ibid., pp. 13-25.
101. Ibid., p. 167.
102. Ibid., p. 15.
103. Ibid., p. 25.
104. Ibid., p. 19.
105. Aratus. 1983. *Phaenomena*.
106. Manilius. 1927. *Astronomica*, p. 31.
107. Ibid., pp. 51-53.
108. Ibid., p. 187.
109. Ibid., p. 27.
110. Ibid., p. 65.
111. Galileo. 1957. *Discoveries and Opinions of Galileo*, trans. S. Drake (Garden City, NY: Doubleday Anchor Books).
112. Manilius. 1927. *Astronomica*, p. 71.
113. Ibid., p. 279.
114. Ibid., p. 7.
115. Ibid., p. 13.
116. Ibid., p. 281.
117. Ibid., p. 279.
118. Orion, R. 1999. *Astrology for Dummies*.
119. Manilius. 1927. *Astronomica*, p. lv.
120. Ibid., p. 35.
121. Ibid., p. 9.
122. Ibid.
123. Ibid., p. 75.
124. Ibid., p. xv.
125. Ibid., p. xiv.
126. Seneca. 1969. *Letters from a Stoic* (New York: Penguin).
127. Ibid., p. 15.
128. Ibid., p. 33.
129. Galen, C. 1997. *Galen: Selected Works*, trans. P.N. Singer (Oxford: Oxford University Press), p. viii.
130. Galen. 1968. *On the Usefulness of the Parts of the Body*, trans. M. Tallmadge May (Ithaca, NY: Cornell University Press).
131. Galen. 1979. *On Prognosis*, trans. V. Nutton (Berlin: Akademie-Verlag), p. 99.
132. Ibid., p. 97.
133. Galen, 1997, *Selected Works*, p. ix.
134. Ibid.

135. Ibid., p. 30.
136. Galen. 1979. *On Prognosis.*
137. Galen. 1997. *Selected Works*, p. xi.
138. Hippocrates. 1923, *Writings*, vol. I. "Air, *Water, Places.*"
139. Galen. 1997. *Selected Works*, p. xxxiv.
140. Galen. 1968. *On the Usefulness*, Book Six.
141. Paracelsus. 1999. *Essential Readings*, trans. N. Goodrick-Clarke (Berkeley, CA: North Atlantic Books).
142. Galen. 1929. *On the Natural Faculties*, trans. A.J. Brock (Cambridge, MA: Harvard University Press), p. 15.
143. Ibid., p. 67.
144. Ibid., p. 69.
145. Ibid.
146. Ibid., p. 71.
147. Ibid., p. 73.
148. Cramer, F. H. 1954. *Astrology*, p. 45.
149. Ptolemy, C. 1998. *Almagest* (Princeton, NJ: Princeton University Press).
150. Copernicus, N. 1995, *On the Revolutions of Heavenly Spheres* (Amherst, NY: Prometheus).
151. Crowe, M. J. 1990. *Theories of the World*, p. 45.
152. Kuhn, T. S. 1977. *The Essential Tension* (Chicago: Chicago University Press), pp. 21-23.
153. Ptolemy, C. 1976. *Tetrabiblos* (North Hollywood, CA: Symbols and Signs) p. 1.
154. Ptolemy, C. 1998. *Almagest.*
155. Ptolemy, C. 1976. *Tetrabiblos*, p. 2.
156. Ptolemy, C. 1998. *Almagest*, p. 104.
157. Ptolemy, C. 1976, *Tetrabiblos*, p. 3.
158. Ibid.
159. Ibid., p. 4.
160. Ibid., p. 7.
161. Ibid., p. 10.
162. Ibid., p. 13
163. Firmicus, M. 1973. *Mathesos: Ancient Astrology: Theory and Practice*, trans. J. R. Bram (Park Ridge, NJ: Noyes Press).
164. Tester, S. J. 1999. *Western Astrology*, p.134.
165. Firmicus, M. 1973. *Mathesos*, p. 1.
166. If two or three constellations were 60° or 120° apart in the sky, they were considered to have special meaning and influences on earthlings.
167. Orion, R.1999. *Astrology for Dummies.*
168. Tester, S. J. 1999. *Western Astrology*, pp. 46-49.
169. Ibid., p. 46.
170. Ibid., p. 47.
171. Firmicus, M. 1973. *Mathesos*, p. 116.
172. Ibid., pp. 87-90.
173. Neugebauer, O. and van Hoesen, H. B. 1959. *Greek Horoscopes*, p. 185.
174. Ptolemy, C. 1998. *Almagest.*
175. Debus, A. G. 1970, "Harvey and Fludd: The Irrational Factor in the Rational Science of the Seventeenth Century," *Journal of the History of Biology*, 3, 81.
176. Harvey, W. 1993. *On the Motion of the Heart and Blood in Animals*, trans. R. Willis (Amherst, NY: Prometheus Books).

Part 2

Medicine in the Middle Ages

3

Theory and Practice

All of the foregoing establishes the astronomical underpinnings of medieval medicine as it gradually evolved through antiquity and into the early Middle Ages. This system of medicine is generally known as Galenic medicine but it is obvious that many thinkers and practitioners were involved in sculpting the form medicine took in the Western World. There were always conflicting views though the basic scheme was the same.[1] The cosmology of Plato and Aristotle, along with the medicine of Hippocrates and Galen, were the forces that shaped medieval medicine and this was not to change until after the Renaissance when the impact of the Enlightenment was first felt.

Macrobius Ambrosius

Macrobius Ambrosius (c. 400 C.E.) was a man about whom little is known. He may have been a Roman official in Spain and Africa, though this is uncertain.[2] Whether he was a pagan or Christian is also unclear. He was well acquainted with Greek and Roman pagan writers and one of the first polymaths to provide an overview of the seven Liberal Arts, though his was admittedly, a sketchy exposition of these subjects. Cicero's *Scipio's Dream* is the basis for Macrobius' *Commentary*.[3] Cicero's treatise is a brief discourse on the soul and its immortality. He was a follower of Plato and believed the human soul emanated from the world soul, having no beginning nor end. Cicero also emphasizes the need for loyalty to the "commonwealth." Initially *Scipio's Dream* was part of a longer work, *De re publica*,[4] patterned after Plato's *Republic*. Scipio Africanus, the Younger, was the adopted grandson of Scipio Africanus who conquered Hannibal in the Punic War of 202 B.C.E. During a dream, Cicero has the younger Scipio transported high above the Earth by both his father (also Scipio Africanus) and grandfather, during which the grandfather enlightens Scipio the Younger, on the soul and his duties to the commonwealth. Macrobius expands Cicero's ten-page work into a 168-page commentary on a variety of topics, including astronomy, harmony, and medicine.

He defines five types of dreams.[5] Cicero believed dreams could predict future events. These soporific insights, Cicero maintains, come directly from the heavens. Macrobius follows the cosmology of Plato's *Timaeus*,[6] including the four elements of Empedocles. Macrobius asserts that the "Creator of the Universe bound the elements together with an unbreakable chain." Earth and fire were so "repugnant" to each other that they required air and water to bind them together.[7] In this way, "the Creator harmonized them so skillfully that they could readily be united." Again, we find the theme of cosmological harmony. He reiterates the concept that each element has two qualities: earth is dry and cold; water, cold and moist; air, warm and moist; and fire, warm and dry. Earth and water are bound together by their coldness; air and fire by their warmth.[8] Water is likewise united to air by its moistness. In this way, all four elements are connected by their neighboring element—earth to water, water to air and air to fire. Additionally, earth is connected with fire because of their mutual dryness. The four elements have different densities and weights and these differences are the same for each. Earth and water differ as water and air and air and fire differ in the same manner as the other elements. This provides a kind of harmony of one element in relation to the others.[9] Macrobius also claims that there are three "interstices" connecting each element. Between earth and water there is "Necessity," so named because clay (earth and water) is the stuff of which bodies are made. The interstice between water and air is "Harmony" and that between air and fire, "Obedience." These are, obviously, more metaphysical than real.

Macrobius is a true Pythagorean and his cosmology is not only one harmonious whole, but it is in numerical harmony as well. He is especially captivated by the number seven. "It is, one might almost say, the key to the Universe."[10] As a consequence, he finds seven almost everywhere in his system. The four elements with their three interstices add up to seven. Thus, the entire sublunary, material world is composed of and united by seven according to Macrobius.

Macrobius' anatomy is also defined by the number seven. "This number marks the members of the body."[11] There are seven viscera: tongue, heart, lungs, liver, spleen, and two kidneys. He ignores the fact that there are two lungs. The organs that receive and expel food and air have seven members as well: pharynx, esophagus, stomach, bladder, and the three parts of the intestine (duodenum, ileum, and colo-rectum).[12] There are seven "tissues" in the body: marrow, bone, sinew, vein, artery, flesh, and skin. The "visible" members are the head, trunk, two arms, two legs, and the "generative organ." And so goes Macrobius' anatomy lesson.

The World-Soul, Macrobius maintains, is constructed out of seven numbers. This was called the "lambda diagram." It is in the form of a Greek upper case lambda: $\wedge$. At the apex is the number 1. Along the left arm are, 2, 4, 8 and along the right arm 3, 9, 27. These are the squares and cubes of 2 and 3; seven numbers in all and since human souls emanate from the World-Soul, our souls must be based on these seven numbers as well. He also recalls the Ancients' claim that "life without air is not sustained beyond the seventh hour and without food beyond the seventh day."[13] Both estimates are incorrect.[14] Macrobius ends his anatomy and physiology lesson by saying that the number seven "is the regulator and master of the whole fabric of the human body.[15]

Figure 3.1
Lambda Diagram

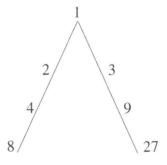

Macrobius is not an inveterate astrologer. He quotes Cicero as calling:

> Jupiter that brilliant orb, so propitious and helpful to the human race and Mars, the ruddy one, dreaded on Earth.

He notes that there are "those who believe that good and evil come to mortals from the planets." He continues by quoting Ptolemy as having said that there are certain harmonic ratios that exist among the planets and this harmony accounts for planetary influences.[16] Harmony is a numbers game for Macrobius. He contends that the Sun and Moon "are the principal guardians of our lives." When they are "favorably aspected," that is, in harmony with Jupiter and Venus, this bodes well for us. Since Saturn and Mars are not generally in harmony with the Sun and Moon, they are considered baneful rather than beneficial for humans.

He goes on to remind us that Plotinus (205-270 C.E.), the Neo-Platonist, says:

> That the power and influence of stars have no direct bearing upon the individual [human] but that his allotted fate is revealed to man by stations and direct and retrograde motion of the seven planets.[17]

Thus, we "obtain premonitions of good and evil from them" but they do not cause good and evil. Macrobius devotes a good deal of space to the topic of musical harmony but this will be covered later.

It is evident from the above that Macrobius believes in the unity and harmony of the Universe. We, along with the Universe as a whole, are connected to the Universe by an unbreakable chain—a harmonious unity. He does not follow Ptolemy and others in promoting a deterministic astrological system. As we shall see next, this makes room for free will in day to day decisions and, therefore, admits of moral behavior.

Augustine of Hippo

Augustine of Hippo (354 - 430 C.E.) is a "Father of the Church"[18] who attempted to "Christianize" the writings of the Ancients, especially Plato. Aristotle was largely lost to the Medievals until the twelfth century.[19] As the Roman Empire slowly disintegrated, their educational system also fell into ruin. Plato was studied and, to a lesser extent, Aristotle. As the Christian Church expanded, it became increasingly apparent that the writings of the Ancients were often at odds with the teachings of the Church. They had to be edited and reformulated. The tenets of paganism were a major influence on the thought of the Church Fathers, as well as, lay Christians of the time, many pagan ideas permeated the fledgling Church, resulting in a tug-of-war between these two religious and philosophical forces.[20] Plato's work was not so difficult to align with Christian theology. His "Good" could easily be equated with the Christian God. His "Intermediaries" became the angels. Aristotle's concept of the "Unmoved Mover" was more of a problem. This "Force" (God for Aristotle) was transcendent and impersonal. It had not created the material Universe. That which provided motion for all things had existed from all eternity, as had the material world. Thus, God and the Universe persisted, side by side, eternally from the past and similarly into the future. This was an impersonal force that set things in motion but did little afterwards. Obviously, this did not describe the providential, anthropomorphic God of the Bible.

Augustine was one of the thinkers of the early Middle Ages, who attempted to bridge this and other doctrinal difficulties. Though fascinated by astrology,[21] he developed a vigorous polemic against this pseudo-science.[22] He notes that the history of the Roman Empire was "neither fortuitous nor fatal." Events occur as a result of a certain divine order and they are neither set for the individual at the time of birth nor subject to prediction beforehand. The will of God does not represent fate in any sense, because humans, by their nature, possess free will. There is no "celestial necessity"— the stars neither cause nor predict future events, only God has prescience of all future events. However, Augustine[23] admits that the stars, "have indeed received a certain power from God…that His commands are fulfilled by them (the stars) instrumentally." As a Neo-Platonist, Augustine believed that angels carry out the tasks God has given to them. This is an extension of the idea that stars, as divine beings, have influence over the Earth and its creatures. This is simply a Christianization of the Ancients' cosmology, but differs somewhat from the astrology of the Greeks and Romans—a system that Augustine finds untenable. It seems that Augustine has only changed the names of these celestial beings. Their functions remain the same, although he did not attribute creative powers to angels, as some Ancients had. He puts much effort into proving that astrology is in error. One of the arguments he uses is medical.[24] He asserts that twins are born (and conceived) at the same time but that their health and life are often very different. Thus, though the position of the stars is the same for both at birth, their medical histories may vary greatly. If the stars were in control, this would not be the case. He specifically denounces "hydromancy" (predictions made by reading water patterns) and "necromancy" (predictions made by communicating with the dead).[25]

Augustine Christianizes several concepts inherited from the Ancients. One example is his view that humans are:

Enlightened from the heavens…a certain intelligible light…illuminates them (humans) that they may be penetrated with light and may enjoy perfect happiness."[26]

This light comes from God and affects both the stars/angels, as well as us humans. Here is an echo of the Aristotelian "ether" that activates the four elements, making us the beings that we are. He also speaks of, "the soul of the world"[27] —this concept taken from Plato's "World-Soul." In his system, Augustine does not specifically mention the four elements but rather refers to water and earth (moisture and dust)[28] as the elements out of which humans are made. Related to this, he adopts the concept of "breath" (the element air?) using the biblical statement from Genesis that God breathed life into the soul of Adam.[29] He seems to be speaking of the "pneuma" of old and possibly relates it to the divine "ether" that ultimately comes from God. Augustine takes away some of the heaven and health connections of the Ancients in rejecting astrology, but he adds and Christianizes others so that they can be easily adopted by the physicians of the Middle Ages and provide a basis for their medicine. With Augustine's scheme, the stars are angels and carry out God's commands. Now, however, the stars are not divine, as Plato claimed, nonetheless they maintain a position of power and are in control of much of what happens on Earth. Galen's system is not denied and neither are the principles that support it. One other point to be made is that astrology was not dead, even though, after Augustine, an effort was made by the Church to suppress this discipline. It certainly was less evident in the early medieval period but during the High Middle Ages and, especially during the Renaissance, the astrologer-physician was once again "alive and well."

A concept, if not introduced by Augustine, expanded upon by him, was that of the first (original) sin of Adam and Eve. Augustine proclaims that death (and by implication disease) is the "punishment of sin" for both evil and good persons.[30] The idea of the gods punishing humankind for impiety toward them is an ancient one. Augustine christianizes this concept, making all "miseries" and "suffering" a result of Adam and Eve's original sin, which has been passed from generation to generation via the father's "seed." Augustine viewed sexual intercourse as intrinsically sinful. Original sin was transmitted from father to his sons and daughters through the "sin of sex." The sexual taboos of the medieval Church emanated from this Augustinian theology and these taboos are found in many theologies today. Disease and death are "penal" in nature, just as punishment in Hell is, except that the latter is eternal. Beginning with the early Middle Ages, a spiritual aspect was added to the concepts of disease and death. There was still harmony involved, for sin was disharmony and "blessedness," harmony with God. Thus, the heaven and health relationship is maintained but in a Christian context.

Spiritual Healing

From Antiquity, magical treatments have blended with medical remedies. Epidemics were unexplained in both ancient and medieval societies. Mist from swamps, intervention of the gods, comets, poisoning of water by Jews and conjunction of certain planets were all presumed causes of plague. Magic and later religious interventions were offered as ways to prevent or terminate pestilence. Sin was the ultimate reason why God allowed disease, thus, amulets, incantations, religious metals, images of saints and rosaries, all remnants of ancient, even prehistoric magic, were offered to ward off the ills of men and women. In the Middle Ages, in no small part due to Augustine's influence, the Church developed many such spiritual aids for preventing the spread of epidemics and healing the sick. The sacrament of "Extreme Unction" (Last Anointing), now known as "The Sacrament of the Sick," was given to those who were dying. The saints became mediators between God and the afflicted. A saint was, in effect, deified by cult followers for their perceived power to protect against or cure a host of diseases. Epidemics were often devastating events in past ages. The plague of Thucydides, which struck Athens in 430 B.C.E., is one of the most famous and its cause still remains unknown.[31]

Justinian's plague that infested Constantinople in 541 B.C.E. is the first known occurrence of bubonic plague, which was to threaten civilization into the nineteenth century.[32] This "pestilence," which devastated Europe (1348-1350), was labeled the Black Death, the name coming from its most frightening manifestation—a dark purple-black, generalized rash due to bleeding into the skin (*purpura*) caused by a clotting disorder associated with bacteremia (blood poisoning). The causative bacillus, *Yersinia pestis*, overwhelms the body's coagulation system and extensive bleeding ensues. Its course was often rapid with some dying within hours of first developing symptoms. There was no treatment and during the epidemic of 1348-1350, it is estimated that 30 percent of the European population died. St. Sebastian has been the patron saint and protector of plague victims since the fourteenth century. This saint was shot with multiple arrows during the Christian persecution of the late third century under the Emperor Diocletian, but miraculously, he survived. His multiple wounds were likened to the many miseries associated with the plague and, thus, the connection was established. Since there was no treatment, only spiritual measures could be employed, making prayers to the saint very popular. Another saint invoked during the plague was St. Roch who was afflicted with this disease. There were many saints whose intercessions were sought during epidemics or with any illness. Prayers to St. Paul were often aimed at curing the sick.

Saints Cosmas and Damian were the most important patron saints of medicine and surgery in the Middle Ages. Cosmas and Damian were physicians (and brothers) who originally came from Arabia. They were Christians who practiced medicine without charge to their patients and were reputed to have performed many cures.

After their death, Emperor Justinian is said to have prayed to them during an illness; he was miraculously healed. Justinian built a church in their honor at Constantinople and the brothers were ensured a permanent place in the realm of spiritual healing. Over the centuries, cult-followers have attributed miraculous cures in the name of their favorite saint. And the practice continues today—even modern medicine has its limitations. The mediation of saints when disease threatens or strikes is a Christian adaptation of more ancient rituals. Instead of the many gods of the pagans, the faithful pray to the saints. Whether it is the gods or saints in the heavens, it is believed that healing could come from above, thus restoring heavenly harmony and harmony of body and soul.

Martianus Capella

Martianus Capella's (c. 425 B.C.E.) best-known work is *The Marriage of Philology and Mercury*[34] deals with the seven "Liberal Arts." This work was widely read in medieval universities.[35] In *The Marriage*, Philology, bride of the god, Mercury, has seven bridesmaids, each of whom personifies one of the seven Liberal Arts. As each is introduced, she explains her "art" and in the process gives an encyclopedic exposition of it. All the gods of Olympus are present at the wedding; each bridesmaid makes her presentation to them. The "maiden of the sky," Astronomica, is the most beautiful of the maidens (the stars are the most beautiful and harmonious of divine beings). In his system, Capella follows Heraclites, assigning heliocentric orbits to Mercury and Venus.[36]

> Now Venus and Mercury, though they have daily risings and settings, do not travel around the Earth at all, rather they encircle the Sun in wider revolutions.

Centuries later, Tycho Brahe is to use the same arrangement of the Solar System, that is, Mercury and Venus revolve around the Sun and the Sun around the Earth.[37] The bridesmaid, Astronomica, describes Apollo (Phoebus) as he drives his chariot and team of blazing horses (the Sun) swiftly through the sky. Apollo was the Sun god and the god of medicine. He was also the god of music, of which more will be said later. Astronomica speaks of the "planetary deities" along with various stars and constellations. Using such metaphors, she lays out the skies for the young, medieval students of astronomy, including those who will soon become physicians. The planetary deities "determine man's destinies" and, though Capella generally minimizes astrology, these concepts are scattered throughout this otherwise purely astronomical work. Capella, through Philology's bridesmaid, describes Jupiter as "health–giving." Jupiter was considered a good sign of health, if it was in the astrological "house" of health when a child was born. The lesser deities (the stars) are composed of an "ethereal" nature.[38] Astronomica claims to have been kept in the "sanctums" of Egyptian priests for 40,000 years, reflecting the perceived antiquity of Egyptian astronomy.[39] Following Hippocrates and Galen, Capella comments on Astronomica's presentation by saying, "Has your choler made a poet out of you?" here speaking of yellow bile and the personality associated with it.[40] It is also mentioned that the planets are associated with certain human characteristics. Saturn, for example, is paired with melancholy.[41]

Capella ends his exposition of the seven Liberal Arts, with Harmony. This will be discussed at length when dealing with music and medicine in a later chapter. Suffice it to say, Harmony and music filled the Universe as Pythagoras claimed centuries earlier. Minerva notes that:

> The maidens (seven Liberal Arts)…have zealously guarded the secrets privy to the divinities…and these maidens bear testimonials of your (the gods') intimate relationship with mortals; for in the cleavage that exists between the divine and mortal realms, they alone have always maintained communication between the two.[42]

In other words, the Liberal Arts bring to humans knowledge that is divine in nature. It is through this communication that harmony connects the gods with mortals:

> Harmony…alone, above all others, will be able to soothe the cares of the gods, gladdening the heavens with her song and rhythms.[43]

It is clear that only Harmony can dispel the quarrels that so often disrupt divine unity and it is only she who can bring harmony to humans, providing health and happiness.

Capella claims that "with song Amphion brought life to bodies stiff with cold."[44] Even the dead can be revived by Harmony. Disharmony produces disease and death; the restoration of harmony heals both.

Although Capella[45] is not thought to have performed many astronomical observations, he estimated, using calculations made during eclipses of the Sun, that the Moon is one-sixth the size of the Earth. His calculations, are flawed in that he is comparing the circumference of the Earth with the diameter of the Moon! Much of what Capella covers, however, is fairly accurate, such as his 27 1/3-day (sidereal) orbital period for the Moon versus its 29 1/2-day (synodic) period.[46] The modern day figures are 27.322 and 29.531 days respectively. Capella was very close in these determinations and demonstrates that he was a competent astronomer.

Capella mentions, in his section on "Harmony," that Medicine and Architecture were standing in the wings "among those ready to perform." This is an allusion to the fact that at one time medicine and architecture were to have been included among the Liberal Arts but were never formally entered into this august group. Nonetheless, medicine in the Middle Ages was intimately associated with the seven Liberal Arts and anyone entering upon a medical career could only do so after "marrying" (mastering) Philology and her seven "bridesmaids." Much of medicine was based in natural astrology but judicial astrology became ever more evident in the late Middle Ages. It continued to have influence among the nobility and even the ecclesiastical hierarchy. Casting horoscopes and astrological calendars was a source of income for many astronomers.[47]

Capella's *Marriage* is a good example of the connections made between medicine and the heavens, both in terms of stellar influences on earthlings and its emphasis on harmony in the macro- and microcosm. Capella's *Marriage* is superior to Macrobius' *Scipio's Dream* in presenting information about the Liberal Arts and was, as a result, more popular in medieval universities.

Figure 3.2

Element	Quality	Humor	Temperament
Fire	Hot, Dry	Yellow Bile	Cholic
Air	Hot, Wet	Blood	Sanguine
Water	Cold, Wet	Phlegm	Phlegmatic
Earth	Cold, Dry	Black Bile	Melancholic

Fig. 3.2 shows the final theoretical form medicine took entering the early Middle Ages. The elements, qualities, humors and temperaments are all viewed as related.

Isidore of Seville

Isidore of Seville (c. 560-636 C.E.) was bishop of Seville for 37 years. As such, he was the Catholic Primate of Spain. Living in a Visigothic and Arian country, he, nonetheless, extended Catholic orthodoxy. He was a polymath with wide interests who promoted education and the Liberal Arts. His interests included theology, canon law, ethics, liturgiology, history, grammar, cosmology, astronomy, physics and medicine.[48] His best-known work is the *Etymologiae*, which is an encyclopedic work intended to define terminology from many disciplines. This work, by Isidore's own admission, was not original but a restatement of many ancient writings both Christian and pagan.

As was often the case in ancient and medieval times, the boundary between physician and layman was indistinct. Polymaths, such as Isidore, wrote on medical topics though not trained or practicing as a doctor.[49] The Church Fathers, including Isidore, incorporated medicine into their educational programs for young monks not so much to ready them for the practice of medicine, rather to illustrate the wisdom and goodness of God. Secondarily, this brought some degree of respectability to medicine while ensuring that medicine would be taught in the Church-dominated educational system of the times.[50] Religious, rather than scientific or humanitarian motivations, were paramount. As seen earlier, spiritual healing was important in the Middle Ages. Sinlessness (harmony with God) was the path to health of mind and body. Following the Galenic system, though somewhat simplified, emotions were anatomically localized: joy in the spleen, carnal love in the liver, knowledge in the heart and anger in bile. These emotions could lead to sin (disharmony with God), which in turn, caused an imbalance in the humors, resulting in disease or even death.

Most monasteries had herbal gardens and some of the monks practiced medicine, at various levels of proficiency, for their fellow monks, often ministering to the local people as well.[51] The practice of medicine by the clergy became problematic for the Church by the thirteenth century and restrictions on "medical monks" were imposed over time. Ultimately no clergyman was allowed to practice medicine at any level.[52] Nonetheless, there continued to be a mixing of medicine and religion and Isidore's writings reflect this blend.

Isidore's physical Universe was based on the classical scheme laid down centuries before by the Ancients and later modified by the patristic fathers.[53] The heavens were composed of ether, which was immutable;

Figure 3.3

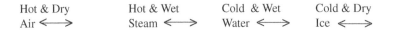

Hot & Dry	Hot & Wet	Cold & Wet	Cold & Dry
Air ⟷	Steam ⟷	Water ⟷	Ice ⟷

the sublunary world consisted of Empedocles' four elements and health was maintained by a proper balance of the four qualities and humors. All of these were united in one harmonic whole. This system was based on speculative reasoning and very little observation went into its construction. That peat (earth) burned to form fire and water evaporated into air when heated, seemed adequate to verify this ancient scheme of things. All four elements were in constant flux—earth to water, water to air and air to fire and back again. That there were inconsistencies in this system seemed not to matter. Peat burned to smoke (air) and then to fire but this process was not reversible. Steam seems to evaporate into air but the reverse process is less evident. The role that the qualities play in this sequence was reassuring for the Ancients. Isidore believed the four elements were in flux with each other and ultimately the solar fire (ether). The heavenly and sublunary worlds were thus tied together in this manner.

The Greeks spoke of the Hyle, which was a formless substance with no qualities of its own but capable of turning into the four elements. Aristotle's "prime matter" would be *Hyle*.[54]

Isidore distributes the elements in the body as follows:

> But flesh is composed of four elements: earth is in the fleshy parts, air in the breath, water in the blood, fire in the vital heat. The elements are mingled in us in their proper proportions of which something is lacking when the conjunction is dissolved.[55]

The vital heat was produced in the heart and was essential to life, according to the Ancients. Isidore confirms that an imbalance in the four elements, and by extension, the four humors and qualities, was the root cause of disease. Aristotle had refined these relations as noted earlier.[56]

In addition to the above associations, fire was aligned with summer, air with spring, water with winter (in the Mediterranean, it rains mostly in winter) and earth with autumn. Also, there was more blood in youth, yellow bile in early manhood, black bile in middle age and phlegm in old age.[57] Acute diseases were said to develop from excess "hot" and chronic diseases from too much "cold." Further, the upper atmosphere, like the fire above it, is calm and clear. The air below this is cloudy and unsettled because of the water in it. Rain comes from this layer of air. The points of the compass are related to the seasons and elements, the winds to the elements and thence to the humors—another sky-Earth connection, noted by Isidore.

When blood was taken from a patient (bloodletting), it would often separate into four layers: the red blood cells at the bottom, related to black bile; just above this may be a lighter, sanguine layer; this clotted fibrin was thought to be phlegm and the serous, clear yellow layer at top, yellow bile. Thus, blood itself contained the other elements.

Hematoscopy involved the visual inspection of blood obtained at the time of venapuncture (bloodletting). Samples were taken as the blood flowed, while clotting, and after it was fully caked. Taste, smell and warmth were the three main characteristics assessed. Diagnosis, therapy and prognosis were all determined from these features. Observation of the blood helped the practitioner determine when to terminate the blood flow. Blood was sometimes strained through a cloth to check for "impurities," which were also believed to be helpful in diagnosis and treatment. It is unlikely this had any clinical value. Several beakers or dishes containing blood samples were used, with which the patient's blood could be compared. Twelve dishes of blood were used to make up to 29 different diagnoses. Hematoscopy was practiced by surgeons, barbers and even bath attendants, all of whom let blood. Blood was considered to be very important as a humor since it was the source of "vital heat."

The *pneuma*, air or breath, was thought to aid in nutrition and facilitated motion. The pneuma was taken in by the lungs, passed to the heart where it became the "vital spirit" or "heat," from there going through the arteries to all parts of the body, including the brain where it became the animal spirit or pneuma psychikon. From the brain, this "psychic air" passed through the nerves to all parts of the body to produce thought and initiate movement. The *pneuma* was thought to reflect the "world pneuma." Isidore denied that the human soul was part of the "world pneuma."[58] Such an association would have had unacceptable theological implications for him—smacking of pantheism.

Isidore of Seville believed in the macro-microcosm relationship, a concept, as we have seen, dating from the time of Pythagoras. Each individual human being was a microcosm reflecting the Universal macrocosm and the latter influenced the former in all aspects of life on Earth.[59] Just as the Universe is reflected in humans, humans are reflected in the Universe. This parallelism, in its various forms, was a major part of medieval cosmology and theology. The individual integrates within him/herself all aspects of universal reality. This concept also provides a crucial link between the material and spiritual worlds—between God and His angelic Intermediaries and the earthly world of mortals. Humankind was, the key to the great cosmic riddle. Understanding human nature provides a way of penetrating the mysterious nature of our Universe. Plato's World-Soul is reflected in the human soul. The Stoics called wo/ man the "little universe."[61] Plato, and Isidore after him, did not believe the human soul was from or part of the World-Soul but simply echoed its nature. Man's[62] reasoning could comprehend only incompletely the nature of the Universe. Still it was this rational part of man that linked us to the Universe as a whole.

Isidore finds anatomical similarities between the human body and the heavens:

> The head refers to the heavens in which are located the two eyes, like the lights of the Sun and Moon. The breath is joined to the air, because just as the breath of respiration is sent thence, so also the blasts of wind come from the air. The belly is compared to the sea, because of a collection of all of the humors, like the gathering together of waters. Finally, the soles of the feet are compared to the [element] earth, since the extremities of the members are dry, or parched, as is also the earth. For truly the mind is located in the eminence of the head, as God is in heaven.[63]

Compared to his other books, in the *Etymologiae*, Isidore's treatment of medicine is brief. He has little on surgery and nothing on midwifery. He briefly mentions amputation, cupping and cautery. His medical definitions are reasonably complete for the times but, like the Ancients, he often views symptoms as diseases—a common practice during the Middle Ages because their failure to understand anatomy and physiology made the grouping of symptoms into specific diagnoses impossible.

Isidore follows the Galenic system, stating that all diseases arise within the body as a result of disharmony among the four humors. Health is the harmony of the humors. The trick in healing is to restore the balance of humors without producing an excess of one or more of the other humors. God does not cause disease but only allows it for His own mysterious purposes. Isidore was aware that rabies came from the bite of a mad dog and so its etiology was outside of the Galenic humoral system.[64]

A few "definitions" from the medical part of *Etymologiae* will suffice to give an understanding of Isidore's approach. He says medicine is:

> That which either protects or restores bodily health; its subject matter deals with diseases and wounds.[65]

His description of the brain is surprisingly accurate:

> The most important part of the body is the head, *caput*,: it has been given this name because all sensation and nerves take their beginning thence, and because every principle of life spring there from. All of the senses are centered there and, in a certain manner, it plays the part of the soul itself, which takes thought for the body.[66]

Regarding the teeth, Isidore comments:

> Gender determines the number of teeth, for they are thought to be more numerous in men, fewer in women.[67]

It is clear that Isidore had never examined a woman's mouth. The *ulna* (the ulna and radius are the two long bones in the forearm), according to Isidore is either an extension of the hand or elbow.[68] This shows a lack of anatomical awareness. The ulna is separate from the hand but articulates with the wrist (carpal) bones while its proximal end articulates with the *humerus* (arm bone) and these, along with the proximal end of the radius, form the elbow. The "pores" of the skin in Latin are called *spiramentum*, i.e., "breathing holes" because the "vivifying spirit is conducted through them (from) outside the body"[69] It was believed that "corrupt air" could enter the body through these pores and cause disease.

Isidore gives the etymological derivation for most of his medical terms. For example, the male *testis* is said to come from the Latin, to testify. Why this association was made is disputed.

Historically, Galen and Hippocrates identified three systems of medicine. Isidore summarizes these. The Empiricists "follow only experience." That is, they observe the patient's symptoms but do not reason to a proper understanding of their cause.[70] "The Methodists study the relationships of neither elements, times, ages nor causes, but only the property of the diseases themselves." In other words, they focus on disease without incorporating other factors into determining etiology, treatment or prognosis. The Logical (dogmatic) practitioner, however, searches "through to their (the disease's) causes in the light of reason" and their cures were then rationally determined. Galen saw his dogmatic approach to medicine as combining both observation and reason, whereas the Empiricists observed without rationally organizing what they saw into a systematic, holistic approach to disease. The Methodists simply used treatments for certain symptoms, cookbook style, without truly understanding what they were treating.

Isidore categorically assigns the cause of diseases to the four humors. "Healthy people are maintained by them and the ill suffer from them. When any of the humors increase beyond the limits set by Nature, they cause illness."[71] Isidore's exposition of Galenic medicine is concise and encapsulates the basic tenets of medieval medicine in an easily comprehended manner, giving a good foundation for later medieval practitioners.

Avicenna

Avicenna (980-1037 C.E.), known as Abu 'Ali al-Husainibn 'Abdallah ibn Sina or simply ibn Sina in the Arab world, was born near Bukhara in Central Asia.[72] He was intellectually precocious and had learned grammar, literature and theology, as well as, the whole of the Qur'an by age ten. Initially ibn Sina studied arithmetic under a vegetable seller (the only teacher of this subject available at the time) but later was tutored in mathematics by Abu 'Abdallah al-Natili, an accomplished astronomer and mathematician. Avicenna mastered the *Almagest* of Ptolemy and Euclid's *Elements* under his tutelage. He also studied jurisprudence and logic followed by physics, metaphysics and medicine. By age sixteen, he had assimilated all the sciences of the day and was well known as a physician. In 997 C.E., at age seventeen, he healed a local ruler and this brought not only fame but also access to the palace library, which contained a large collection of "books." He immersed himself in these works and soon wrote his first treatise (on mathematics) at age twenty-one and subsequently completed a twenty-volume work on all the known sciences. After his father's death, he left Buhkara and led a wanderer's life, frequently moving from place to place, depending on the local political climate. At one point, he was imprisoned for four months because of political problems, only to escape and settle in a more peaceful setting where he could study and write. During this period, he began the construction of an astronomical observatory. His best-known medical work is The *Canon of Medicine*,[73] which is the primary source for what follows.

Avicenna's cosmology contains both Aristotelian and Neo-Platonic elements. Following Plato, he believed that each heavenly sphere had a soul, which accounts for its motions. He speaks of the souls of the spheres, as well as, "Intelligences" which are intermediaries between God and the Universe. These Intelligences could be viewed as angels and the celestial spheres as living beings. This Neo-Platonism is mixed with the Aristotelian concept that all motion in the Universe is due to "desire" on the part of heavenly bodies to "actualize what is potential."[74] He envisioned the motion of the spheres as circular, since this is the "most perfect" of geometric figures, as Aristotle had claimed, many centuries before. Ibn Sina said the luminosity of stars and planets is due to their "nobility of being." The heavenly regions are composed of ether, in contrast to the sublunary region consisting of the four elements. The former is eternal and unchanging (except for location) and, in turn, they give order to the sublunary region. Each celestial sphere has its own "generative intellect." There are nine spheres and each, in turn, generates the sphere below it. These are all contingent souls. The highest sphere is God or "Being Itself" who is necessary and not contingent, in the philosophical sense. Through this series of "intellections," the Universe is created. God remains transcendent in this scheme. Ibn Sina adapted the Platonic system of Forms for his cosmogony. Pure Being (God) remains entirely independent of the world He has created. The ninth sphere ibn Sina calls the "Heaven of Heavens." The first element comes from this sphere— also labeled the "Generative Intellect." The second sphere is that of the signs of the zodiac. Since each sphere impacts the one below it, we can see in this structure the influences that the upper bodies have on earthly bodies.[75] The lower spheres contain the "Intelligences." As one moves down this hierarchy, impurity is introduced until reaching the sublunary world of generation and corruption. Earthly bodies are composed of the four elements but receive their form from the Intelligences.[76] Ibn Sina goes on to explain how the four qualities developed and, from them, the four elements.

For Avicenna, this is a religious cosmology based on angelology. The angels influence the world in many ways and, though their modalities of influence may differ, conceptually the result is the same—the heavens affect what happens on Earth including health and disease.[77] The influencing beings involve both the Intelligences and the Spheres. These beings guide the lives of men and women on Earth. In spite of Avicenna's religious cosmology, he writes in defense of astrology.[78] His acceptance of astrology is incomplete, however, and in various treatises he attacks magic, the occult and predictions of future events. He draws on the Qur'an to support these views, "None in the heaven and on the earth knows the Unseen, save Allah."[79] He explicitly condemns judicial astrology but allows for natural astrology. As with Aristotle, he uses astronomical-medical analogies to explain many of his ideas. For example, he compares the astronomy of the *Almagest* to the anatomy of medicine and Ptolemy's astronomical tables to medical remedies. In addition, though he criticizes judicial astrology, he does not deny the cosmological foundations upon which it is based. The sublunary region receives its very existence from the Intelligences and spheres above. Earthly beings are totally dependent on them and passive in respect to the influences that emanate from them. All events in this world of generation and corruption result from heavenly influences and these influences go beyond the obvious effects of the Sun on the ripening of fruit and the lunar tidal effects. Without these heavenly controls, all would be chaos in the sublunary world. Thus, natural astrology has a place in Avicenna's system.

In contrast to the Intelligences (angels) that have only form and no matter, the sublunary region of change has both. The earthly region is characterized by rectilinear motion rather than the "perfect" circular motion of the heavens. And the sublunary region is made up of the four elements, rather than ether.[80]

> The elements are simple bodies. They are the primary components of the human being throughout all its parts, as well as all other bodies in their varied and diverse forms.[81]

The four elements account for this region's generative and corruptible nature. Ibn Sina follows the Ancients in describing fire as warm and dry, air as warm and moist, water as cold and moist and earth as cold and dry. Other qualities are derived from these qualities; for example, softness comes from moisture and hardness from dryness. The four elements are continually transformed from one to the other. Fire condenses into air and air evaporates into fire etc. This is basically the same structure that Aristotle and Galen had proposed. Avicenna's meteorology is derived directly from Aristotle and is consistent with a natural astrology with all its implications for the heavenly effects on health and disease. The Sun is the paramount factor in this process but the other celestial bodies also play a role.

In *The Canon of Medicine*, Avicenna equivocates concerning the influences of planets:

> To go further, and to agree with the Ancients that epidemics and the like had relation to planetary influences is not necessary; nor is it necessary to dismiss their possibility off-hand. It is not safe to argue that there is no relation between the planets and stars and life on this earth simply because some relation once thought to be true is now discredited. If the whole Universe is one organic whole, there cannot but be some relation.[82]

In Avicenna's view, there is room for the effects of the stars and planets on the health and disease seen in humans, even if these effects are not always easily related to events in our lives. There is, in his opinion, at least a theoretical basis for such a relationship.

Ibn Sina defines three types of disease: "primitive," coming from outside the body, such as trauma and burns; "antecedent," that is, related to the humors and "conjoint" in which he includes blockage of an orifice by a humor and sepsis with fever.[83] He ascribes all diseases to "repletion by humors" and "depletion by humors"; both of which can be traced back to changes in the qualities and elements. Even the "primitive" causes are related to the four qualities. Burns, for example, would be due to an excess of fire.[84] It is unclear how trauma fits into this scheme. He states that an individual's temperament, which is due to his or her most prevalent humor, determines how one is affected by disease.[85] If the climate and season are "harmonious" with the person's temperament then s/he will tend toward health. For example, if ones temperament is hot and dry (cholic) then he or she will, presumably, do well in a cold and wet season, such as winter. Ibn Sina suggests that phlegmatic persons are more prone to epilepsy, paralysis and apoplexy (stroke) in a cold season.[86] A choric individual is prone to delirium, mania, acute fevers and acute inflammatory swelling in a hot season. Ibn Sina puts great stock in meteorology, as Aristotle had. There are, of course, certain diseases that tend to occur at certain times of the year, though they are not necessarily due to temperature or moisture.

Avicenna is arguably the greatest of medieval physicians. His works were widely read and used extensively in emerging medieval medical schools. Like Galen, he was an astute diagnostician and impressed his patients with both his erudition and clinical acumen. Demeanor was everything in the practice of medicine since therapies were so often ineffective. The physicians of note during Antiquity and the Middle Ages had to have charisma, an air of confidence, wide knowledge of the Ancients and a discerning diagnostic ability. It also helped to be a prolific writer on medicine. Avicenna was all of these.

Moses Maimonides

Moses Maimonides (1135-1204 C.E.) was born in Cordova, Spain, son of a rabbi. One of his teachers may have been the famous Arabic physician and philosopher, Ibn Rushd (Averroes) (1126-1198). Whether Averroes actually taught Maimonides is in question but certainly he was influenced by this physician-philosopher. Maimonides was schooled in both theology and philosophy and at age twenty-three wrote a treatise on the Jewish calendar, indicating an early interest in astronomy and mathematics.[87] In time, he studied medicine and practiced this art for most of his life, though always maintaining an interest in theology and astronomy. Maimonides was altruistic in his medical care, spending much time treating the poor. He wrote a treatise on psychology, *The Eight Chapters*, but the work most read today is *A Guide for the Perplexed*, which contains elements of theology, philosophy, astronomy and medicine.

His expertise in medicine was highly prized and he was offered a position as court physician to the King of the Franks in Ascalon but elected to take a post as physician to the Visier of Saladin, King of Egypt.[88] While in his employ, he wrote a treatise on hygiene. He describes himself as a "conscientious and exact person." His duties to the King were very time consuming and his practice busy, leaving little time for study and writing. After his work at the palace each day, he faced an "antechamber filled with Jews and Gentiles, nobles and common people awaiting my return."

Though Maimonides was basically an Aristotelian, he denied the eternity of the Universe. He maintained that only what can be grasped by ones intellect, perceived by his senses or was based on good authority, could be trusted. As a consequence, astrology was rejected *out right*.[89]

In chapter LXXII of The *Guide for the Perplexed*, he draws a parallel between the Universe and man

> Know that the Universe in its entirety is nothing else but one individual being; that is to say the outermost heavenly sphere together with all included therein, as regards individuality is beyond all question a single being.... The variety of its substances—I mean that sphere and all its component parts—is like the variety of substances of a human being.[90]

He goes on to say that just as humans are composed of flesh, bone, sinews and various humors, so too, the Universe is composed of the spheres with the Earth at the center. There are the four elements of earth, water, air and fire with the ether surrounding all these. The Earth is encircled by water, water by air, air by fire and ether is beyond fire.[91] His cosmology is Aristotelian, though the idea of a living Universe is Platonic, as we have seen. The number of spheres he suggests is at least eighteen, possibly more (Aristotle posited fifty-five). The spheres each possess a soul, as Plato had suggested 1,500 years before. All sublunary substances are composed of the four elements in varying proportions and are subject to change, generation and destruction. One element can be transformed into another: fire condenses into air, air into water and water into earth. The reverse also occurs. This process is compared to the recurring positions of the stars and planets in the sky as they come and go across the heavens. "All the spheres revolve with constant uniformity." He was apparently unaware of the variable velocities of the planets known since Antiquity and which had forced Ptolemy to devise his complex system of epicycles and equants.

In another passage Maimonides asserts:

> Again, the principle part of the human body, namely the heart, is in constant motion and is the source of every motion noticed in the body; it rules over the other members and it communicates to them through its own pulsations the force required for their own functions. The outer most sphere by its motion rules in a similar way over all other parts of the Universe and supplies all other things with their special properties. Every motion in the Universe has thus its origin in the motion of the spheres; and the soul of every animated being derives its soul from the soul of that same sphere.[92]

The forces that emanate from the spheres to the sublunary world include those that combine the elements into minerals and other objects as well as the vegetative forces found in plants; the vital force of every living being and the force that provides intellectual function.[93] Along with Aristotle, Maimonides believes in spontaneous generation of life from dunghills, presumably engendered by the heat of the Sun.[94] He also compares the four humors and elements to the fifth element as both essential features of their respective spheres—super- and sublunary.

Maimonides says, "The same forces that operate in the birth and temporal existence of the human being operate also in his destruction and death." He further explains that since the vital functions of the body, such as digestion and secretion, are not intelligent but operate blindly, it is this irrational element, which may lead to excesses or deficiencies of humors, thus causing disease. He goes on to say:

> The same forces that organize all things and cause them to exist for a certain time, namely, the combinations of the elements which are moved and penetrated by the forces of the heavenly spheres that same cause becomes throughout the world a source of calamities such as devastating rain, showers, snow storms.... malaria and other catastrophes by which a place....or even a country may be laid waste.[95]

He implies that natural disasters, such as earthquakes and plagues, result from celestial influences. He notes that the disorders of digestion and secretion can lead to the absorption of humors that are too hot or too cold, too thick or too thin and thus result in diseases like "scurvy, leprosy, cancer or elephantiasis." There is in his scheme an implied linkage between the heavenly forces and the forces in humans which, when disordered and disharmonious, cause disease.

Maimonides affirms the concept of humans as microcosms, just as the Ancients had. This analogy, in his view, applies only to the intellectual function of human beings, so that dumb animals cannot be considered microcosms.[96] Although he follows earlier writers concerning the macrocosm-microcosm, Maimonides stops short of making direct connections between the divine, intellectual heavenly bodies and the diseases of humankind. The cause of disease follows from the "irrational" nature of the elements, as described above. He draws a parallel between the Universe as a whole and "individual men," stating that there is a "complete harmony" between the two.[97]

Other concepts of the Ancients, such as Pythagoras' universal harmony, are included in Maimonides' writings but he does not carry them as far as his predecessors. The idea of harmony in the Universe, however, does admit of a certain connection between heaven and Earth and a relationship between the stars and sickness. With regards to herbal remedies, he notes that, "There is no single herb below without its corresponding star above that bears upon it and commands it to grow."[98] Each individual herb has its own individual star and is influenced by this star. He goes on to say that

> Although the influences of the spheres extend over all beings, there is besides the influences of a particular star directed to a particular species; a fact noticed also in reference to the several forces within one organic body.

He ties the Moon to water, noting the connection of the Moon to the tides. There is also the influence of the Sun on fire. Just as these celestial objects affect water and fire so, too, the planets influence the atmosphere. It is worth noting here that Maimonides adopts eccentric orbits for the planets and rejects Ptolemy's epicycles—a concept anticipating Kepler's elliptical orbits by 500 years.[99] The influences of the stars are at a distance and do not imply any direct contact with earthly objects. Distance and even time do not constrain these influences, according to Maimonides.

Furthermore, though critical of astrology, he uses many of the same concepts that connect astrology—at least natural astrology— to medicine. It was easy enough, then, for later physicians to resurrect astrological medicine and allow for the direct effect of stars on both diseases and therapies, as was the case in the Elizabethan period. From the foregoing, it is evident that Maimonides follows the Ancients in most respects with minor variations. He was undoubtedly most influential in forming the medicine of the later Middle Ages. His approach was balanced and reasoned in spite of the limitations imposed on him by the state of science in which he found himself.

The Medieval Medical School

Education in late Antiquity up to the early Middle Ages was based on the seven Liberal Arts; a system introduced by the Greeks and adopted by the Romans.[100] The term "liberal" is said by Tester to be derived from the "arts" studied by "free" (*liber, -era, -erum*) men in early Greek culture. Others interpret the term as derived from the Latin *liber, -eri* meaning book, because this educational system was based on studying the classic books of Antiquity. By the sixth century, c.e., as noted earlier, the Liberal Arts had been divided into two parts: the *Trivium*, which consisted of grammar, rhetoric and dialectic and the *Quadrivium*, containing arithmetic, geometry, music and astronomy. The *Trivium* was the elementary stage (and thus the word trivial) and prerequisite to the study of the other four disciplines. Grammar meant Latin grammar. Rhetoric included figures of speech, forms of oratory, metrics and literary devices. Dialectics was the study of Aristotelian logic from the *Prior Analytics*.[101] The Quadrivium was little studied in Antiquity and the early Middle Ages. What we know as arithmetic, educators at the time called *algorism*, which meant calculations on the abacus. Arithmetic dealt with numbers, including the configurations made from them. For example, 3 square is depicted as 3 rows of 3 dots, which form a square geometric figure.[102] This, undoubtedly, was Pythagorean in origin and represented a kind of numerical harmony. Such shapes fascinated the Pythagoreans. The tetraktys was the most discussed of such figures and was composed of ten dots that formed an equilateral triangle. [103]

Figure 3.3
The Tetraktys

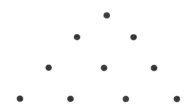

(Fig. 3.3) Things *are* numbers, according to Pythagoras and the arithmetic of the Middle Ages was an offspring of this idea. Augustine of Hippo echoes this idea when he says, "You (God) have ordered all things in number.[104] Geometry included elementary Euclidian concepts, as well as, "geography," which described the Earth with all its lands and seas. Music dealt with principles of harmony rather than instrumental or vocal arts. This was again Pythagorean and related in part to the harmony, not only in the Universe, but also between the macrocosm and microcosm. These are concepts clearly tied to the medicine of the times. Both harmony and musical modes had healthy and unhealthy effects on a patient's soul and were linked to the theory behind physical and psychic disorders. More will be said of this later. Astronomy came under the headings of the Latin, *Astronomia* and *Astrologia*.[105] These terms were often used interchangeably, though in the *Quadrivium*, astronomy was more astronomical than astrological. Although astrology was still popular among noble wo/men and the common people, it was much less so in educated circles. Early in the fifth century C.E., the philosophers Boethius and Martianus Capella were prized for their astronomy but later Ptolemy and Aristotle came into vogue. Sacrobosco was the most popular astronomical authority studied through much of the late medieval period.

John of Hollywood or Johannes de Sacrobosco (c. 1200-1250 C.E.) is most famous for his astronomical manual, *Sphere*, which was the standard astronomical text for much of the late Middle Ages. Any student of the Liberal Arts was familiar with this work. Not much is known of Sacrobosco except that he was probably an Englishman and that he taught at the University of Paris.[106] The *Sphere* includes material on the general structure of the Universe, the celestial spheres, phenomena caused by the daily rotation of the heavens, planetary motion, theories of the Sun and Moon as well as an explanation of eclipses. Sacrobosco also wrote a treatise on time reckoning. These texts were probably written in the early thirteenth century and remained popular through the fourteenth century and were studied in all major universities of Europe, including Cambridge, Montpellier and Paris.

By the thirteenth century, medieval universities had developed from cathedral schools to stadium *generale* or "universities" with four major faculties: Arts, Canon Law, Medicine and Theology. To enter one of the latter three disciplines the student had to have completed the basic curriculum and obtained a Masters of Arts degree. The Faculty of Medicine was not, strictly speaking, a "Faculty of Science." Science, as such, was studied within the seven Liberal Arts, especially the *Quadrivium* as detailed above.[107] Science came under the heading of "Natural Philosophy," which was based largely on the Aristotelian model and included basic botany, anatomy, physiology and embryology as found in Aristotle's[108] *On the Generation of Animals* and Galen's[109] *Natural Faculties*. In 1255 C.E., the University of Paris authorized all of Aristotle's works so that these became standard texts including *De Coelo*[110] and *De Meteorlogica*.[111] His cosmology is found mainly in *De Coelo* and the elements of "natural astrology" in *De Meteorologica*. Those studying law or theology were tonsured clerks, that is, on a track leading to ordination to the priesthood. This was not the case for medical students who were almost always laymen. The fourth Lateran Council in 1215 C.E. had prohibited priests from practicing as physicians.[112] The university student studied mathematics, as related to *Computus*; that is, the determination of the date for Easter each year. Numbers, according to Pythagoras, provided a way of describing nature in mathematical terms. Aristotle vehemently denied that numbers could be "forms," as he defined forms, so these mathematical ideas were minimized in the Middle Ages but the concept of harmony and the relationship of the heavens to the lives of Humans persisted, especially in medicine.

Sacroboscos's astronomical instrumentation was limited, as best we can tell, to the quadrant and sundial or *horologium*, so that his observational astronomy was rudimentary. His one mathematical work was the *Algorismus*, which dealt with geometry, and was used to provide the basic mathematical underpinnings for astronomy. Sacrobosco did not emphasize Aristotle, displaying more interested in Euclid's geometry. He used Ptolemy very little because the *Almagest* was generally beyond the grasp of the *Quadrivium* student. He was aware of precession[113] and celestial coordinates,[114] as well as, the latitude of the Arctic Circle (23° 51' N). Sacrobosco knew how to determine the time it took for a zodiac sign to rise completely above the horizon, offering evidence for his interest in astrology. In addition, he laid out the seven "climates," which had been so important for the Ancients in explaining such human characteristics as skin color and temperament. Sacrobosco saw the science of astronomy as partly *naturalis* and partly *mathematica*, providing a link between mathematics and natural philosophy.[115] Scholars of the Middle Ages referred to it as *scientia media* or a middle science—a discipline bridging demonstrative mathematics and observational natural sciences. As a consequence, Sacrobosco used astronomy in a much broader pedagogical sense than we do today. It was, for him, a vehicle for "smuggling" in material from diverse disciplines that could then be taught to his students. It provided a fundamental tool to introduce the student to a wide range of topics. For the medical student, astronomy was not only the basis for the study of the human body and its functions, but also the foundation for medical practice. Diagnosis and therapy were, to varying degrees, dictated by the heavens. So, astronomy not only provided a broad platform from which a wide range of topics could be discussed but it also allowed the student-physician an understanding of the etiology and therapy of diseases. The heavens explained diseases in an age when bacteria, viruses, metabolic disturbances, neoplasms, and the like were unknown.

The medieval university, as it developed, offered increasing legitimacy to medical practitioners and allowed them to distinguish themselves from barbers, apothecaries and surgeons. They developed their own "livery" or distinguishing robes, became respected "physiks" and by the time of James I, had been granted a royal "medical monopoly."[116]

Hildegard of Bingen

Hildegard of Bingen (1098-1179 c.e.) was one of the most talented thinkers of her time.[117] She was a visionary, mystic, healer, linguist, poet, artist, musician, playwright, biographer, theologian, preacher and spiritual advisor to nobles and ecclesiastics alike. Her main medical work, *Physica,* contains remedies derived from plants, trees, stones, fishes, birds and other sources. In the twelfth century, the term physics, as it had in Antiquity, meant "medicine" and a "physik" was a healer or physician. Her book is often entitled, "Book of Medicinal Simples"—a "simple" being a medicinal plant or remedy derived from it—not combined with other herbs. She often spoke of her treatments as "subtleties" which refers to secret powers hidden in natural creatures by the "Divine" for use by humans. Her theology is Roman Catholic in type but God was in the heavens and worked through intermediary angels. We have seen this scheme before in the writings of Augustine and others. There is a parallel here between the "Spheres and Souls" of the Ancients which were also intermediaries between God and humans. She connects humans with the heavens as follows:

> O man look to man for man has the heavens and earth and other created things within him. He is one, and all things are hidden within him.[118]

This is her restatement of Pythagoras' macrocosm-microcosm dyad.

She advocated a Galenic system with diseases and cures linked to the four "powers" or qualities—hot cold, dry and moist. Diseases arise from an imbalance of these qualities and therapy is aimed at restoring their normal balance.[119] In some instances, she claims that "like cures like" so that an imbalance of cold would require an herb that was "cold." The rationale behind this was that "cold" draws out excess "cold" from the body. On the other hand, she might use the "opposite cures opposite" rule, so that an imbalance of "cold" would require a "hot" herb to replace the excessive "cold." Humors were also central to her medical theory. In the traditional Greek humoral theory, yellow bile is hot, blood is dry, phlegm is moist and black bile is cold. Hildegard varied this theme slightly, borrowing from Eastern medicine, in speaking of dry, damp, foamy, and cool. Any imbalance of these qualities caused disease and restoration of the imbalance brought health. As you will recall, the hot, cold, dry, and moist are linked cosmologically to the elements of fire, air, water and earth and, thus, to heavenly, ethereal influences.

In the *Physica*, Hildegard lists each remedy as hot or cold and those diseases it will cure. Wheat is hot; it is good for both the healthy and the sick, providing flesh and blood. If bran is removed from wheat, the wheat is "weaker" and produces more "mucus" in the person and in this form the herb is not good for sick persons.[120] Whole wheat, however, is good in treating someone with an "empty brain....vexed by delusions," that is, an insane person. The grains of wheat, after cooking, are wrapped around the head of the patient and the "brain will be invigorated" and the patient made whole again. Cooked wheat, Hildebrand asserts, is also good for backaches, and dog bites. Nutmeg "has great heat" and will "open up your heart" and "diminishes all harmful humors." She provides therapies for everything from dropsy (heart failure) to leprosy, though leprosy in the Middle Ages could mean any type of chronic dermatitis. Herbs were often graded from one to four degrees according to how wet or dry, hot or cold they were. An example of this is found in *The Medieval Health Handbook*, otherwise entitled *Tacuinum Sanitatis*:

> Oranges: The pulp is cold and humid in the third degree, the skin is dry and warm in the second. Their candied skin is good for the stomach. They are difficult to digest. (but this can be neutralized if) accompanied by the best wine.[121]

Hildegard devotes a chapter to the elements of fire, air, water and earth.[122] Air "near the Moon and stars wets the heavenly bodies." This air is compressed within the bodies of animals but when they die, air leaves them and reverts to its original state. This view of air is reminiscent of the *pneuma* described by the Ancients. Water is offered as a treatment for eye problems. It was commonly held that vision was a result of the eyes sending "fiery" rays out to objects seen.[123] As "fiery," the eyes when inflamed or dry, could be helped by applications of cool water. She also discusses the specific uses of waters from the sea, the Rhine, Moselle, and other rivers. Each had a role in her practice. Earth is "naturally cold and has many powers in it." It is cold on the surface especially in the winter because the Sun draws its powers back from the earth at this season.[124] She asserts:

> The earth shows its greenness in heat (from the Sun), its dryness in cold. In winter the Sun over the earth is sterile and drives its heat into the earth, so the earth can reserve its various grasses. Through heat and coldness, it brings forth all grasses.[125]

Here she affirms the influence that the Sun has on earth and its changes from season to season. This system seems rational enough, but the herbalist's premises are then carried beyond what we would now consider scientific conclusions, relying on speculative reasoning as employed by the Ancients. For the physicians of these early times, however, it made logical sense and provided a theoretical basis for their art.

Hildegard speaks of different types of earth such as calamine "Calamine is neither hot nor cold in due proportion, but tepid."[126] And as a result, diminishes mucus when it is in excess. Although "earths" including minerals, such as calamine, are classically considered cold and dry, she claims the few drops of water in earth allow plants to germinate and grow.

Hildegard's system is typical of the herbalists of her day and these few examples give the reader some idea of the reasoning behind this Galenic system of therapy. It is internally consistent (but not empirically established) if one accepts the astronomical concepts upon which it is based.

Diagnosis, Treatment, and Prognosis

The Book of Secrets of Albertus Magnus is a typical medieval herbal guide but it has a stronger astrological emphasis.[127] Although attributed to the famous thirteenth century philosopher-scientist and teacher of Thomas Aquinas, Albertus Magnus (c.1206-1289 C.E.), it is unlikely that he was the author. *The Book of Secrets* was one of many such treatises that claimed knowledge of ancient mystical, covert therapies known to only a select few. The writing of Hermes Trismagistis, first recorded in the third century C.E., is probably the most famous of these mystery texts and contains furtive facts said to date from ancient Egyptian times.[128] Both these works were popular well into the Renaissance. Included are "secrets" about herbs, stones, beasts and planets. The author of the *Book of Secrets* begins by condoning the "science" of magic, claiming to take his lead from Aristotle. A typical entry concerns the benefits of the herb marigold:

> The virtue of this herb is marvelous for if it be gathered, the Sun being in the sign Leo, in August, and be wrapped in the leaf of a Laurel, or Bay tree and a wolf's tooth be added thereto no man shall be able to have a word to speak against the bearer thereof, but words of peace. And if any thing be stolen, if the bearer of the things before named lays them under his head in the night, he shall see the thief and all his conditions.[129]

Such prescriptions show not only the celestial connections to herbs and how they bring the qualities of the heavenly bodies to the person using them, but also demonstrate the astrological features so often found in these therapies. This treatise is filled with drawings of herbal plants that were, in fact, included in Albertus Magnus' *Naturalia*. The author of *The Book of Secrets* devotes a chapter to the planets. It is essentially an astrological presentation. He supports judicial astrology and includes drawings from *Naturalia* that show the mythical gods associated with each planet.

The *Physica* and *Book of Secrets* are typical but contrasting works on medieval therapies; they both deal with herbal and related therapies but the latter is strongly oriented toward astrological medicine. Hildegard, perhaps because of Church prohibitions against such tendencies, minimizes this aspect of herbal medicine. In either system, the stellar influences are evident—Hildegard echoing Augustine and various ancient pagan writers.

Medical Practice and Practitioners

The medieval approach to diagnosis and therapy focused on individual symptoms rather than syndromes (collection of symptoms).[130] Under this system, a different medicine would be given for each symptom. In a case of pneumonia, for example, one therapy would be prescribed for fever, another for productive cough, a third for chest pain etc. There were a great many therapies used by the medieval physician and the other types of healers of the time. In addition to university trained physicians, there were surgeons, rarely university trained; apothecaries, who sold and used a wide variety of medicines including herbs, minerals, sulfur, mercury even arsenic, learning their trade through apprenticeship; barber-surgeons, generally schooled by a mentor in strictly practical techniques; leeches,[131] who, as the name implies, used leeches in their bloodletting procedures; phlebotomists, specialists in letting blood by surgical means, herbalists, who relied entirely on herbal or related remedies; midwives, treating gynecological disease and assisting at deliveries; and finally there were sage, old women and faith healers providing medical services.[132]

The remedies offered included the herbs and other "medicines" noted above, as well as, strictly surgical procedures, such as incision and drainage of abscesses, amputations and even trephination (boring holes into the skull). Cataract surgery was performed as well.

The astrologer-physician would diagnose and treat, without even seeing the patient using only heavenly signs to provide diagnostic information. Uroscopy (the examination of the urine) was frequently the only "laboratory test" done but much trust was placed in the color, turbidity, smell and even taste of the urine. Urine that was "highly colored and greasy" would indicate an excess of choler. A "feeble color" along with a mucous discharge was associated with too much phlegm. Uroscopy would often allow the physician to diagnose and treat without touching or even seeing the patient.

Clysters (enemas) were a mainstay of therapy. One such clyster used by the surgeon, John of Arderne (fourteenth century), contained water, mallows, green chamomile, wheat bran, salt, honey (or oil), assorted herbs and soap.[133] Purgatives of various sorts were used to "cleanse" the bowels and rid the patient of excess humors. A poultice is a soft, moist mass of bread, meal, clay, or other adhesive substances, usually heated, spread on a cloth, and applied to warm, moisten, or stimulate an aching or inflamed part of the body. Such treatments were aimed at restoring humoral balance. Some "cold" treatments were given in order to keep in the heat that was lacking in the patient or draw out the "cold" that was present in excess. Other healers used "hot" herbs to add heat to the patient who was thought to be lacking in this quality. The theory was, as stated previously, based on the "elements" and their related qualities.

In addition to the above remedies, diet, exercise and abstinence from unhealthy drinks, such as alcohol, were often prescribed. Alcohol was thought to cause gout, flatulence and hemorrhoids (all of which are true). Such programs, during times of plague, were believed to keep the pores of the skin closed to "infected air."[134] The idea of infected air was not, of course, based on microbial theory but rather considered to be air from the disturbed atmosphere, again relating the heavens to disease. Moses Maimonides had suggested that the planets, because of their retrograde motion, stirred up the air in the atmosphere, creating winds that could bring disease.[135] Warm and moist foods, such as chicken and almonds were often served to the medieval invalid, since these foods were considered most akin to the ideal humoral state. They helped to replenish depleted humors.

As with the Ancients, climate and weather were thought to play a major role in the cause and cure of disease. Dutch women, as one example, were thought to bear more females than males. Humid winds, which often brought rain to Holland, were considered more favorable to the conception of females. Women were thought of as cold and wet as opposed to men who were viewed as warm and dry. The north winds that seemed to cleanse the air of "unhealthy vapors" were judged more masculine.[136] A certain chauvinism is evident in these theories and date from the time of the Ancients.

The heart was regarded by Aristotle as the principal organ of the body, and contained a "spirituality" related to the *pneuma* or vital air mentioned earlier. Again, this *pneuma*, though not specifically tied to the ether, bears an implicit relationship to the stuff of which the stars are made. Circulation was not understood until Harvey's work on the subject,[137] however, the Ancients believed that the blood flows back and forth within the arteries and veins. This rhythmic, to and fro motion corresponds to the rhythm and harmony found in the heavenly spheres. The pulse, which resulted from this alternating motion, was considered an important diagnostic tool. It was also a useful guide to therapy.[138] To a lesser extent, examination of the feces and blood was used in medieval medicine. Color, heat, texture and smell were all part of the "laboratory" testing of these specimens.

Thus, the physician, having talked to the patient, examined him or her to the extent that decency would allow, inspected the urine and possibly blood and stool, sometimes casting a horoscope, was then ready to proffer a diagnosis and embark on a course of therapy aimed at re-establishing the humoral balance. It is not the purposes of this book to cover in any detail either diagnosis or therapy over and above what has already been said about these procedures. The theory behind diagnosis and therapy and how it relates to astronomy and universal harmony is our primary focus here.

Finally, astrological medicine in the Middle Ages requires a second look. In 1348, Phillip VI of France requested that the medical faculty of the University of Paris give an opinion on the cause of the Black Death. [139] It was the opinion of these physicians that:

> An important conjunction of three higher planets in the sign of Aquarius, which with other conjunctions and eclipses, is the cause of the pernicious corruption of the surrounding air.[140]

They went on to note that the conjunction of "Mars and Jupiter causes great pestilence." According to their theory Jupiter, which was a warm and humid planet draws up evil vapors and Mars, which is hot and dry, sets fire to these vapors. Mars was considered a malevolent planet generating both choler and wars. A physician at Montpelier medical school suggested that there were "extraterrestrial rays" that accounted for the pattern of spread of the plague throughout Europe.

Augustine of Hippo had condemned astrological forecasts. Other theologians of the Middle Ages, such as Isidore of Seville, were more comfortable with investigating man's relationship to the stars.[141] Albertus Magnus and Robert Grosseteste, also a thirteenth-century theologian, made a clear distinction between natural and judicial astrology. In their view, natural astrology could be used by sailors to predict weather and by doctors to cure diseases. Nicolas of Orsme and Phillipe de Meziéres, in the next century, laid down the "legitimate" limits of medical astrology. Specifically, doctors were not to make predictions about future events. This was considered contrary to the teachings of the Bible. These views, however, allowed latitude in the use of astrology in diagnosis and therapy. Charles V, in 1371, called for a joint faculty of astrology and medicine at the University of Paris. Many nobles were fervent believers in astrology, both natural and judicial.

The belief that each zodiac sign ruled certain anatomical parts of the body persisted throughout the Middle Ages. The use of Galen's critical days in the gathering of herbs, bloodletting, administering of purgatives, timing of surgery, even the cutting of hair and nails was still prevalent in the late Middle Ages. The presence of the Moon in a certain "house" in the sky that ruled over a given part of the body, made treatment of that portion of the anatomy dangerous or even potentially fatal. When the Moon, for example, was in Aries, procedures on the head were proscribed. Some thought that the best day for treating dropsy by bloodletting was 17 September.[142] The same procedure for migraine was best done on 3 April. The "Dog Days" of summer were considered particularly unlucky—"Dog Days," of course, relating to the presence of Sirius, the dog star, in the sky.

The harvesting of herbs was often determined by the heavens.[143] Not only time, but also the place and manner of picking herbs were thought critical to their ultimate efficacy. One mandate required, that a young child pick a certain herb in late August. Another advised waiting until the Moon had entered the "house" of Virgo before cutting marigold. The purity of soul of the herbalist's assistant played a role as well. Unless the assistant who picks the herb is sinless, the herb would be ineffective. Timing was everything. For example, only if Jupiter was in the "ascendant" (rising just before the Sun) at the time of picking the herb, nothing could be done to preserve the "virtue" or curative power of the herb. Such recipes might include the saying of several "Our Father's or "Hail Mary's" as well.

The "sphere of Pythagoras,"[144] a circular chart attributed to the famous astronomer-mathematician, was used in the Middle Ages to predict the outcome of an illness. This involved numerology as well as the day of the lunar cycle when the patient first became ill. These prognostications were considered useful even if they forecast impending death, for it allowed the stricken patient to confess his or her sins before dying, thus assuring admission to heaven.

The astrolabe was employed to determine the exact day, hour and even minute for the administration of medicines or the performance of surgery. Some professors of medicine such as Pietro d'Ahano, who taught astrology, philosophy and medicine at both Paris and Padua, complained that many practitioners determined the time of therapy without due regard for details—they were sloppy in their astrological calculations. In the late Middle Ages and into the Renaissance, many healers were astrologer-physicians such as Paracelsus and Robert Fludd, of whom we shall say more later.[145] The University of Bologna medical faculty, in 1445, stipulated that all medical students study astrology for four years. Neither Oxford nor Cambridge universities promoted astrology, however.

Paradoxically, as medicine moved into the Enlightenment, more emphasis was given to the astrologer-physician while, at the same time, medical giants such as William Harvey, came on the scene. Often the two types of physicians practiced side-by-side. Robert Fludd, as noted above, was an astrologer-physician but also a friend of Harvey's and an advocate of Harvey's explanation of human circulation.[146]

Notes

1.   Crombie, A. C. 1995. *The History of Science from Augustine to Galileo*, vol. II (New York: Dover), p. 25.
2.   Macrobius. 1990. *Commentary on the Dream of Scipio*, trans. W.H. Stahl (New York: Columbia University Press), p. 6.
3.   Ibid., pp. 67-77.
4.   *De re publica*: Concerning the State (literally the public thing).
5.   The five types of dreams are (1) the enigmatic; (2) prophetic; (3) oracular; (4) the nightmare; and (5) the apparition.
6.   Plato. 1977. *Timaeus and Critias*.
7.   Macrobius. 1990. *Commentary*, p. 105.
8.   Ibid.
9.   Ibid., p. 106.
10.   Ibid.
11.   Ibid., p. 115.
12.   Ibid., p. 116.
13.   Ibid.
14.   Without air, brain death occurs in less than seven minutes; without food, one dies within several weeks—around five or six—but this varies. Without water, death ensues within two weeks. In older or sicker patients, death may come in five days.
15.   Ibid., p. 117.
16.   Ibid., p. 167.
17.   Ibid., p. 168.
18.   Augustine is arguably the most important Catholic theologian.
19.   Emperor Justinian (485-565 C.E.) closed the Aristotelian and Platonic schools in Athens in 529. After this Simplicius (d. 549) wrote several commentaries on Aristotle's works (*On the Physics*, 1992, Syracuse, NY: Cornell University Press, for example) but in the West few could read Greek and until the Arabs translated Aristotle's works four/five centuries later and transmitted them to Western Europe, Aristotle was essentially unknown there.
20.   Armstrong, K. 1993. *A History of God* (New York: Ballantine), pp. 37-39.
21.   Pope, H. 1961. *Augustine of Hippo* (Garden City, NY: Image Books), p. 86.
22.   Augustine, St.. 1950. *City of God* (New York: Random House Modern Library), pp. 142-144.
23.   Ibid., p. 43.
24.   Ibid., p. 144.
25.   Ibid., p. 240.
26.   Ibid., p. 305.
27.   Ibid., pp. 121-122.
28.   Ibid., p. 436.
29.   Ibid.
30.   Augustine, St. 1950. *City of God*, p. 413.
31.   Marks, G. and Beatty, W.K. 1976. *Epidemics* (New York: Charles Scribner's Sons), p. 19.
32.   Ibid., p. 44.
33.   Capella, M. 1977. *Martianus Capella and the Seven Liberal Arts*, trans. W. H. Stahl & B. L. Burge (New York: Columbia University Press).
34.   Tester, S. J. 1999. *Western Astrology*, p. 103.
35.   Capella, M. 1977. *Martianus Capella*, p. 333.

36. Grant, E. 1996. *Planets, Stars, and Orbs: The Medieval Cosmos*, 1200-1687 (New York: Cambridge University Press), p. 39.
37. Capella, M. 1977. *Martianus Capella*, p. 317.
38. Ibid., p. 318.
39. Ibid., p. 316.
40. Ibid., p. 331f.
41. Ibid., p. 347.
42. Ibid., p. 349.
43. Ibid., p. 352.
44. Ibid p. 334.
45. The sidereal period of the Moon's revolution around the Earth is measured by the stellar background, whereas the synodic period is the time between two successive new Moons. Because the Earth is revolving around the Sun this time is longer.
46. Casper, M. 1993. *Kepler*, trans. and ed. C. D. Hellman (New York: Dover), pp. 340-342. Kepler cast horoscopes for the nobility.
47. Isidore of Seville. 1964. *Isidore of Seville: The Medical Writings* (Philadelphia: American Philosophical Society), p. 7.
48. Ibid., p. 11.
49. Ibid., p. 15.
50. Ibid., p. 17.
51. Kneel, E. 1966, "Medical Practice by Clergy: the Prohibitions of Canons 159, s 2 and 985, 6° of the Code of Canon Law" (Rome: Canon Law Dissertation). The problem for the Church was that medicine was taking the clergy from their monastic duties and prayers and there was concern that celibates were treating women.
52. Isidore of Seville. 1964. *Isidore of Seville*, p. 23.
53. Ibid., p. 23.
54. Ibid.
55. The diagram of the four elements is based on one in Isidore of Seville's *Liber deresponsione mundi*, Augsburg, 1472, Original in the Huntington Library.
56. Ibid., p. 24.
57. Ibid., p. 25.
58. Ibid.
59. Ibid., p. 26.
62. "Man" is used here because neither Plato nor Isidore considered women capable of rational thought in the philosophical or theological sense.
63. Ibid.
64. The idea of contagion slowly developed though the centuries, but was not to be accepted until bacteria were discovered and connected to disease in the 19th century.
65. Ibid., p. 55.
66. Ibid., p. 40.
67. Ibid., p. 42.
68. Ibid.
69. Ibid., p. 55.
70. Ibid.
71. Ibid.
72. Nazr, S. H. 1978. *An Introduction to Islamic Cosmological Doctrines* (Boulder, CO: Shambhala), p. 177.
73. Avicenna. 1930. *The Canon of Medicine*, trans. C. Gruner (London: Luzac & Co.).

74. Nazr, S. H. 1978. *Islamic Cosmological Doctrines*, p. 237.
75. Ibid., p. 203.
76. Ibid., p. 206.
77. Ibid., p. 237.
78. Ibid., p. 238.
79. Ibid., p. 239.
80. Ibid., p. 241.
81. Avicenna. 1930. *Canon of Medicine*, p. 34.
82. Ibid., p. 56.
83. Ibid., p. 173.
84. Ibid., p. 175.
85. Ibid., p. 184.
86. Ibid., p. 184.
87. Maimonides, M. 1956. *The Guide for the Perplexed*, trans. M. Friedlander (New York: Dover), p. xvi.
88. Ibid., p. xvii.
89. Ibid., p. xxv.
90. Ibid., p. 113.
91. Ibid.
92. Ibid., p. 115.
93. Ibid., p. 116.
94. Ibid.
95. Ibid., p. 117.
96. Ibid.
97. Ibid., p. 118.
98. Ibid., p. 164.
99. Ibid., p. 167.
100. Tester, S. J. 1999. *Western Astrology*, p.101.
101. Aristotle 1984, Prior Analytics, *The Complete Works of Aristotle* (Princeton, NJ: Princeton University Press).
102. Tester, S. J. 1999. *Western Astrology*, p.102.
103. Guthrie, K. S. 1987. *Pythagorian Source Book*, p. 29.
104. Augustine, St. 1950. *City of God*, p. 401.
105. Tester, S. J. 1999. *Western Astrology*, p. 103.
106. Pedersen, O. 1985, "In Quest of Sacrobosco," *Journal of the History of Astronomy*, 16, 175.
107. Ibid.
108. Aristotle. 1942. *Generation of Animals*, Loeb Classics, trans. A. L. Peck (London: Harvard University Press).
109. Galen, C. 1929, *On the Natural Faculties*, trans. A.J. Brock (Cambridge, MA: Harvard University Press).
110. Aristotle. 1984. "De Coelo."
111. Aristotle. 1984. "Meteorology."
112. Kneel, E. 1966. "Medical Practice."
113. Precession is the gradual shift of the Earth's axis over a 26,000-year cycle so that the direction the axis points to forms a circle in the sky with the "north star" varying over time, always returning to Polaris. This is why Sirius was a summer star for the ancient Egyptians but is a winter star for us today.
114. Celestial coordinates are like longitude and latitude but are called right ascension (longitude) and declination (latitude) when applied to the sky (celestial globe).

115.   `Pedersen, O. 1985. Sacrobosco.
116.   Woolley, B. 2004. *Heal Thyself: Nicholas Culpeper and the Seventeenth-Century Struggle to Bring Medicine to the People* (New York: HarperCollins), p. 36.
117.   Bingen, H. 1998. *Physica*, trans. P. Throop (Rochester, VT: Healing Arts Press)
118.   Rawcliffe, C. 1999. *Medicine and Society in Later Medieval England* (London: UK: Sandpiper), p. 33.
119.   Bingen, H. 1998. *Physica*, p. 5.
120.   Ibid., p. 10.
121.   Arano, L. C. 1996. *The Medieval Medical Handbook: Tacuinum Sanitatis*, trans. O. Ratti and A. Westbrook (New York: George Braziller).
122.   Bingen, H. 1998. *Physica*, pp. 99-104.
123.   Park, D. 1997. *The Fire within the Eye* (Princeton, NJ: Princeton University Press), p. 39.
124.   Bingen, H. 1998. *Physica*, p. 102.
125.   Ibid.
126.   Ibid., p. 103.
127.   Best, M.R. and Brightman, F.H. 1999. *The Book of Secrets of Albertus Magnus* (York Beach, ME: Samuel Weiser).
128.   Billings, A. 2000, Corpus Hermeticum, http://www.hermetic.com/texts/index.html.
129.   Best, M.R. and Brightman, F.H. 1999. *Book of Secrets*, p. 4.
130.   Rawcliffe, C. 1999. *Medicine and Society*, p. 59.
131.   The label "leech" could apply to any type of practitioners.
132.   Siraisi, N. G. 1990. *Medieval and Renaissance Medicine*, pp. 18-20.
133.   Ibid., p. 61.
134.   Ibid., p. 40.
135.   Maimonides, M. 1956. *Guide*, p. 165.
136.   Rawcliffe, C. 1999. *Medicine and Society*, p. 41.
137.   Harvey, W. 1993 *On the Motion of the Heart and Blood in Animals*, trans. R. Willis (Amherst, NY: Prometheus Books).
138.   Galen, 1997, *Galen: Selected Works, The Pulse for Beginners*, trans. P.N. Singer (New York: Oxford University Press), pp. 325-344.
139.   Gottfried, R. S. 1983, *The Black Death* (New York: Macmillan Free Press), p.110.
140.   Rawcliffe, C. 1999. *Medicine and Society*, p. 82.
141.   Ibid., p. 85.
142.   Ibid., p. 88.
143.   Ibid., p. 98.
144.   Rawcliffe, C. 1999. *Medicine and Society*, p. 100.
145.   Ibid., p. 90.
146.   Debus, A. G. 1970. "Harvey and Fludd: The Irrational Factor in the Rational Science of the Seventeenth Century," *Journal of the History of Biology*, 3, 81.

4

Music and Medicine

"There is a Charm: a power that sways the breast;
Bids every Passion to revel or *to rest*;
Inspires with Rage, or all your cares dissolves *in air*;
Can sooth Distraction, and *alone dispel despair*.
That Power is Music!"[1]

In view of the belief that the Universe is one harmonious living being and that music resounds throughout the celestial spheres, it is not surprising that music found a place in the sublunary world of earthlings. Music was quickly tied to the four elements, qualities, humors, and temperaments and, as a consequence, was linked to health and healing. The association of music and medicine has its roots in prehistory and evidence of its antiquity is with us today in the healing rituals of contemporary primitive peoples.[2] The beat of drums to heal the sick is still heard around the world. In Greek antiquity Apollo, who was the god of both arts, symbolized the bond between music and medicine.[3] Asclepius, his son and personification of the medical role of Apollo, was a later mythological development that emphasized the affiliation of music and medicine. The Hippocratic Oath begins:

I swear by Apollo, Physician, by Asclepius,
By Health, by Panacea and by all the gods and goddesses.[4]

Some evidence for a music-medicine bond has been presented above. In this section, specific aspects of music will be covered to more fully define this association.

Pythagoras

As we have seen, Pythagoras (sixth century B.C.E.) and his school at Croton are noted for their mathematical formulations; the most famous is the Pythagorean theorem.[5] It is also well documented that the mathematical basis of music was established at Croton.[6] Using the "monochord," an instrument with but one string, Pythagoras identified the classic harmonic ratios. This, arguably, is the most important musical discovery ever, and set in motion the study of harmonics for the very first time. Pythagoras was trained in Egypt as a healer and became an advocate of music as a healing art. He was one of the first to speak of harmony as fundamental to the workings of the Universe, viewing the cosmos as the "macrocosm" and each human as a "microcosm." The human body and soul were a reflection of this universal harmony. Human harmony was seen as the essence of health. Plato advocated music as one element in a "healthful place."[7] Aristotle, though less specific in connecting music and medicine, believed that music could both soothe and excite the emotions, providing a catharsis just as if the patient had received medical treatment.[8] In Rome, dance and song were considered to have salutary effects.[9] Cicero believed in the healing power of dancing and singing as a medicament for the soul.[10] Galen was of the same opinion.[11] Herophilus (c. 335-c. 280 B.C.E.), an Alexandrian physician, is said to have determined the health of a patient by the rhythm of his arterial pulse.[12] Cassiodorus (sixth century C.E.) noted the spiritual benefit of musical training and its influence on both our physical and moral lives.[13]

Boethius (c.460-524 C.E.) agreed with Plato that the human soul was conjoined with the *anima mundi*[14] and when the *anima humani* is in harmony with the universal soul, it has a soothing effect on both soul and body.[15] The medieval doctor often described (as Galen had[16]) the pulse in terms of musical proportions and musical verse.[17] According to Pietro d'Abano, the rhythm of the pulse is dactyls in infancy and iambs in old age.[18]

Pythagoras was the most important of the Ancients who contributed to our understanding of music. His famous monochord was the "research instrument" that revolutionized the field of musical theory and it is necessary for a fuller understanding of this discipline to briefly review his work in harmonics. [19]

Fig. 4.1
The Pythagorean Monochord

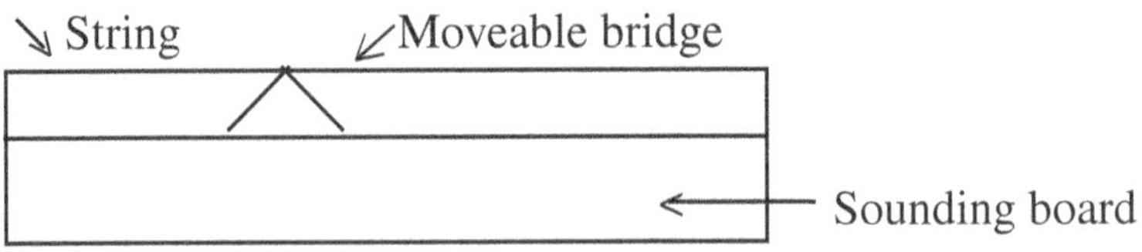

In experimenting with the monochord, Pythagoras found that if the whole string vibrates after being plucked, without the bridge in place, this represents the "fundamental" tone of the string. The shorter the string, the higher the vibration frequency (pitch) of the string and the longer the string the lower its pitch. If the bridge is placed so that the string is effectively divided in half, the frequency of vibration of the two halves is exactly twice the fundamental frequency. Similarly, if the string is divided into thirds, each of the three segments will vibrate at exactly three times the fundamental and with each division of the string, there is a proportional change in vibration frequency—a string 1/4 as long as the original, vibrates four times as fast; 1/5 as long, five times as fast and so on. In other words, there is a reciprocal relationship between this ratio and its fundamental.

Pythagoras, in describing these musical-mathematical relationships, found it easy to understand the Universe as one great harmonic system. By extension, he not only believed that the Universe was a harmonious system, but that:

> The Nine Muses were constituted by the sounds made
> by the seven planets (and) the sphere of the fixed stars.[20]

Pythagoras believed that there was music throughout the Universe, although humans could not hear this music, either because our ears were incapable of doing so or we were so used to hearing it that it was no longer evident to us. In terms of his medicine, Porphyry (a biographer of Pythagoras) claims Pythagoras, "soothed the passions of the soul and body by rhythms, song and incantations." Porphyry goes on to suggest that Pythagoras was one of very few who could actually "hear the Harmony of the Universe and understood the universal music of the spheres." There were believed to be eight to ten crystalline spheres, which controlled the motions of the stars and planets, including the Sun and Moon and that each of these spheres had its own harmonic music. Just as the macrocosm is a harmonic being[21] so too is the microcosm. Thus, the soul and body are healthy if in harmony with the Universe, diseased if discordant with this cosmic harmony.[22]

Music in Greek and Roman Medicine

Not all the Ancients supported Pythagoras' views on harmony and healing. The Greeks were the first to introduce "rational" medicine to the Western World.[23] They wanted to move away from a supernatural, mythical explanation of the physical world to a natural, empirical description of the phenomena that surround us. Hippocrates (or his school) writes:

> For if a man by magic and sacrifice will bring the Moon down, eclipse the Sun and cause storm and sunshine, I shall not believe that any of these things is divine, but human, seeing that the power of the godhead is overcome and enslaved by the cunning of man.[24]

In other words, the gods cannot be tricked or enticed into healing anyone simply by human incantations. This can only be accomplished through natural means since diseases, like eclipses, are natural phenomena.

Greek intellectuals, including physicians, did not believe in myth and magic.[25] For them "medical song" (incantations) was superstitious, magical instruments not suited to "rational medicine." They did, for the most part, believe in the ancient view of the Universe as a harmonious system, even believing, perhaps, that there was a kind of celestial music permeating the heavens. The use of therapeutic music was employed by some Greek healers, like Pythagoras, as noted above.[26] Caelius Aurelianus tells of a piper who played songs over parts of the body in "which quivering and throbbing were relaxed after the pain had been destroyed."[27] Theophrastus, the heir to Aristotle's school of philosophy (the Lyceum), reported that a flute player could relieve gouty arthritis with soothing music.[28] Snakebites were also said to be cured by flute music "if played skillfully and melodiously." Democritus, the atomist, claimed (*On Deadly Infections*) that many ills could be cured by music. The connection between body and mind was so close that music, which calmed the soul, could do as well with the body. Caelius Aurelianus, however, writes that, "Soranus (a Greek physician) asserts that those men were very stupid who believed that the strength of the illness can be expelled by melodies and songs."[29] Diocles believed that incantations were nothing more than "friendly consolation." In other words, being with a patient and talking to him or her would do as well as music. In general, the ancient Greek physician rejected incantations. In the Hippocratic treatise *The Sacred Disease*, it is suggested that incantations for epilepsy are offered as a treatment simply because it is a way for musicians to make money.[30]

Galen also rejects incantations as not medically useful.[31] The Romans were of a similar mind. Both Celsus and Varro warn against the use of incantations and the Roman government did not consider men that used incantations "true" physicians. Galen states:

It is not a learned physician who sings incantations over
patients which should be cured by cutting.[32]

Even Homer derides the use of incantations.[33] Some Greeks, however,
admitted the difficulties associated with not using incantations in treating
their patients. Even Plato saw their use as deeply ingrained in the minds
of the common person.[34] For many Athenians, disbelief in incantations
meant disbelief in the gods—the same kind of impiety that doomed
Socrates. Hippocrates makes this point in *The Sacred Disease*.[35] Greek
physicians, dedicated as they were to the god, Asclepius, found it difficult
to abandon incantations. But Pliny claims that most Greek and Roman
physicians had discarded incantations.[36] Eudoxus, physician-astronomer
and colleague of Aristotle, nonetheless, supported magic[37] as a valid discipline, according to Pliny. In contrast to what Plato says in the *Laws*, Pliny
claims Plato taught magic after learning it abroad.[38] Pliny does support
the claim that Democritus was given to the use of magic, in the form of
incantations. He also reports that Druid doctors used magic, presumably
incantations, in their practice of medicine. Pliny is one of the sources for
the Roman ban on medical incantations.[39] Related to incantations is the
whole question of religious music as it was used in the medieval Church.
This will be covered later, but suffice it to say that Hippocrates did not
deny the use of religion in medicine.[40] That there was harmony in both
the macrocosm and microcosm was a generally accepted concept among
the Ancients. It was also widely held in medical circles that an imbalance
in this harmony related to disease but the use of incantations seemed too
magical to be truly scientific. Undoubtedly the common Greek or Roman
held views contrary to the intellectuals of the time. There was, obviously,
a mixed attitude toward music therapy among the Ancients. The use of
music as healing therapy, however, did not go away.

Martianus Capella's Theory of Harmony

Martianus Capella's (fifth century C.E.) *Marriage of Philology and
Mercury* [41] deals with the seven Liberal Arts. The last chapter of this
treatise tells of Harmony, a personification of one of the Liberal Arts.
Capella joins medicine to Harmony in this section of *The Marriage*. First,
medicine and architecture (two of the bridesmaids at the marriage) are to
perform together. However, Jupiter, who is master of ceremonies, defers
their performances because both deal with "mortal subjects and their arts
are concerned with mundane matters" whereas Harmony resides with
the "celestial deities." Jupiter goes on to say that,

> It would be a grave offense to exclude from this company the one bridesmaid who is
> the particular darling of the heavens.

Capella speaks of Harmony as essential to the structure of the heavens, thus perpetuating the theme of celestial musical harmony.[41] Capella links the heavenly bodies (gods) with mortals through the Liberal Arts:

> For, in the cleavage that exists between the divine and mortal realm, they alone have
> always maintained communication between the two.[42]

The maidens Apollo speaks of in this passage are Genethliace (casting of horoscopes), Symbolice (riddles used in telling the future) and Oeonistice (augury using bird formations). These three "maidens" are connected to the divine heavens because they can do what gods do—foretell the fate of humans. But of the maidens who connect the divine and human worlds, it is the next maiden that is most glorious:

> After them a beautiful maiden will appear,
> radiant in celestial light.[43]

Jupiter then orders Harmony to come forward. She is the last of the maidens to instruct and entertain the gods.

> She indeed, above all others, will be able to soothe the cares of the gods,
> gladdening the heavens with her song and rhythms.

It is implied that Harmony "has rejected mortals and their desolate academics" at some time in the past. She is now willing to restore to them the "melic"[44] arts. Mortals had previously been unappreciative of her instruction in harmony. Capella has already done the same for the other Liberal Arts through *The Marriage of Philology and Mercury*.[45]

There are gods and mortals at the wedding and Harmony "soothes the breasts" of both with her music. Many musicians are among the guests including Amphion,[46] who had:

> Brought life again to bodies stiff with cold, made mountains animate, and gave to
> hard rocks sensibilities, teaching them to follow his refrains.[47]

Capella gives to music not only the ability to raise the dead but animate mountains and rocks as well. It is told how Arion calmed the seas with "his tuneful song" through the aid of Harmony. One by one, Harmony charms the gods, changing their mood to a gentle, loving one. Entranced by song, Cupid lays down his quiver and bow, no longer aggressively shooting everyone in sight. Pleasure and Beauty (personified) join in saying, "Let us sing and let us love." "Harmony's song delights and soothes the spirits of all the gods."[48]

Harmony reaffirms the notion that the celestial bodies produce a harmony concordant with Pythagorean proportions. She describes herself as "the twin sister of heaven" and proclaims she has not forsaken numbers (Pythagorean ratios). She has followed the course of "sidereal spheres…assigning tones to the swiftly moving celestial bodies."[49]

> When the Monad[50] and first hypostasis of intellectual life was conveying to earthly habitations, souls that emanated from their original source, I was ordered to descendwith them to be their governess…introducing restraint and harmony into all things.[51]

This numerical harmony is the "universal law for all mankind." She recalls that Pythagoras had affirmed the "firmly binding relationship between souls and bodies." She taught humans music with cithara[52] and flute and brought music to birds, the rustling of trees and the gurgling of rivers, recalling:

> I have frequently recited chants that have had a therapeutic effect upon deranged minds and ailing bodies; I have restored the mad to health through consonance, a treatment that the physician Asclepiades[53] learned from me. [54]

She tells also of calming a drunken mob with her music and asks, "Have not I myself brought healing to diseased bodies with prolonged (musical) therapy?" She states that the Ancients cured fevers and wounds by incantations. Asclepiades in like manner, cured patients who were "stone deaf." Thales of Crete is said to have "dispelled pestilence" playing the cithara. The maiden goes on to tell of animals that respond to music, even rocks that sing when someone smiles at them. Her message is clear and reaffirms the "wisdom" of the Ancients, especially that of Pythagoras—there is harmony throughout the Universe; this is what keeps it working in an orderly manner and since disease is disharmony, music can restore to health the afflicted body or soul. Capella affirms an ancient system that explains heaven and health as one "logical" matrix. This is not the "rational" approach Greek physicians had promulgated. It is a return to the supernatural and mythical. By the end of the Roman Empire and the rise of Christianity, faith and the supernatural had once again become the guiding principles of society.[55] This was the beginning of church music as the main source of healing music. Incantations once again became a medical medium.

Boethius and Harmony

Boethius, the sixth-century philosopher and theologian, wrote a treatise on music, *De Institutione Musica*, which laid the foundations for the study of music and harmony throughout the Middle Ages and Renaissance.[56] It was the most influential book of its type during this period. Boethius notes:

> The sense of hearing is capable of apprehending sounds in such a way that it not only exercises judgment and identifies their differences, but very often actually finds pleasure, if the modes are pleasing and ordered, whereas it is vexed if they are disordered and incoherent.[57]

As noted above, music was one of the subjects of the *Quadrivium*, along with arithmetic, astronomy, and geometry. All four were considered mathematical disciplines and all were involved in the search for truth. Boethius believed music has a physical effect on the soul. "For nothing is more characteristic of human nature than to be soothed by pleasant modes or disturbed by dissonant sounds." Music extends to every human endeavor. The young as well as the aged are "attuned to musical modes by a kind of voluntary affection." Thus, music is integral to the nature of wo/men and can deeply affect their moods. "None is excluded from the charm of sweet song." He goes on to agree with Plato that "the soul of the Universe was joined together according to musical concord." Further, he asserts that humans "are put together in its (the Universe's) likeness." The harmony of the Universe, including its musical underpinnings, provides the harmony of both body and soul. This must be true because, Boethius reasons, "likeness attracts and unlikeness disgusts and repels." Besides the pleasant and unpleasant aspects of music and its relationship to harmony, which include health and disease as the Ancients claim, there is a moral aspect to music. "A lascivious disposition takes pleasure in more lascivious modes or is often made soft and corrupted upon hearing them." Similarly a "rougher spirit finds pleasure in more exciting modes." He points out that the various modes, such as Lydian and Phrygian,[58] are named after local peoples because they take pleasure in these modes. Again, he agrees with Plato that the introduction of music that is not "chaste and temperate" will defile the character of the people.[59] The Spartans had observed that "chromatic"[60] modes corrupted children. Music can "affect and reshape" the mind. That music can corrupt the youth is a theme present in many ancient and contemporary cultures. Corruption was akin to disease and was seen as a spiritual imbalance—a kind of disharmony. Music has power to affect both body and soul according to Boethius and this includes health and disease. He claims:

It is common knowledge that song has many times calmed rages, and that it has often worked great wonders on the affections of bodies or minds.[61]

He recalls that Pythagoras had calmed a drunken adolescent, excited by a Phrygian mode, by singing a "spondee."[62] The citizens of Lesbos and Ionia are said to have been saved from "very serious illness" through a song.[63] Sciatica was also cured by music. Empedocles (fifth century B.C.E., physician-cosmologist, is reported to have calmed a homicidal youth with music. Music was used to induce sleep and alternately help one wake up in the morning. Boethius also claims Hippocrates treated Democritus with music when he was thought to be mad because he offered an atomistic theory to explain the workings of the Universe. He notes that a mourning woman may cease crying if exposed to sweet music.[64]

Boethius defines three kinds of music: cosmic, human and instrumental.[65] Cosmic music must exist, though unheard by humans, Boethius reasons, because such fast moving celestial bodies as stars and planets have to make some sound. Further, he asserts:

If a certain harmony did not join the diversities and opposing forces of the four elements, how would it be possible that they could unite in one mass and contrivance.[66]

In this passage, Boethius ties together cosmic, human and instrumental harmony. Some force must unite the four elements and it is harmony that seems to be the most rational binding principle. This view is consistent with the theoretical basis of medieval medicine, that is, the balance and imbalance of the elements, qualities and humors account for health and disease. Music is the "glue" that not only holds the Universe together but also provides a rational explanation for health and disease.

Whoever penetrates into his own self, perceives human music.
For what unites the incorporeal nature of reason with the
body, if not a certain harmony and, as it were, a careful tuning
of low and high pitches as though producing one consonance?[67]

If the four elements were not properly united in the body by the harmony of music, this would disturb the qualities and humors, resulting in a diseased mind or body. According to this theory, disordered music would disrupt the musical bonds that hold the elements and humors in proper balance. Harmonious music could restore these bonds, returning the body and/or mind to health.

Boethius was, like Martianus Capella, an advocate of the seven Liberal Arts. He believed the subjects of the *Quadrivium* were basic to an understanding of the Universe. Geometry, arithmetic, along with astronomy and music, were all mathematical sciences and, as such, could bring demonstrative (mathematical) certitude to our understanding of the world. The conclusions arising out of these four liberal disciplines possessed a kind of mathematical infallibility, which made their study essential to our full awareness of the world and the Creator who fashioned all celestial and earthy marvels that daily fill us with delight and awe.

Hildegard of Bingen: Her Music and Medicine

> When, however, the Devil, man's deceiver, heard that he had begun to sing by the inspiration of God and through this would be drawn to remember again the sweetness of the songs of the heavenly homeland, seeing the machinations of guile coming to nothing, he was made frantic.[68]

This statement by Hildegard of Bingen encapsulates the shift in emphasis that had gradually taken place over the last centuries of the Dark Ages. There was still music in the heavens but this was from heavenly choirs of angels. Neo-Platonic and Judaic influences in the early medieval Church had transformed the divine stars of Plato into celestial intermediaries. The spheres were still singing with heavenly harmony but it was the harmony of angels.

Hildegard of Bingen's view of the Universe is similar to the Ancients but with modifications.[69] She emphasizes the concept of "winds" that influence the health and well-being of humans. These winds, which are celestial in nature, affect the workings of body and mind.

> Then I saw[70] that by means of the different qualities of the winds and their concurrent airs, the humors which are in man are stirred up and changed, assuming their qualities.[71]

We note here the reference to both the qualities and humors so basic to medieval medicine. She compares the winds and their effects on humans to various animals, such as the lion, deer, crab or wolf. The humors affected by these winds sometimes "rise up fiercely like a leopard" but at other times are softer like a lamb.

She embraces a macro-microcosmic view of heavenly influences just as Pythagoras had some sixteen centuries before. Heavenly bodies influence the body and soul because they are of a similar (divine) nature. She makes comparisons between the rivers of Earth and the veins of humans.[72] Likewise, the soul, which is airy, is related to the air above. In addition, Hildegard adds a religious spin to all of her cosmology. Virtues, such as humility, hold good works together just as the "nerves"[73] hold the body together.

Additionally, after the Fall, wo/men had lost the angelic voice God had given them in the Garden of Eden. With their expulsion from Paradise and the infirmities they were now subject to, Adam and Eve could no longer bear to hear the "power and sonorousness" of their formerly heavenly voices. God did allow them less magnificent voices and these voices, along with the musical instruments He taught them to play, allowed them to still praise God in psalms and hymns. The lyre mentioned in Psalm 32 has ninety-one lower notes, which are from the body and higher ones that are from the soul. Disharmony is for Hildegard the root of disease of both body and mind. Now, however, the emphasis shifts toward a moral rather than a purely physical cause of disease. The Fall had made disease possible and the Devil was instrumental in the etiological disharmony that underlay all maladies. Hildegard considered music-making a divine process.[74] Thus, only God could give humans harmony. God was the great healer because it was God who provided this healing harmony. Doctors or other healers might be the instruments of healing but God was the source for all cures. It was believed the Devil made no music because he possessed no harmony—he was discord personified. Hildegard saw wo/man united with God as the ultimate harmony.[75] For her, liturgical music was central to this union.[76] God was perfect harmony and only by union with God could we, as humans, achieve perfect harmony of *anima* and *corpus*—perfect health of mind and body. This system provided not only rational medical theory but also theological certitude. It was a rational and religious structure that seemed like a beautifully constructed cathedral—a monument to God. Many of her concepts about God and music came, she claimed, from divine inspiration (her visions). She felt divinely touched—these views came not from her own mind but from the mind of God. As a consequence, they could not be fallacious. This, along with her tightly structured rationalism (as she saw it), made her system one not to be denied.

Hildegard of Bingen represents the medieval Catholic view of health and disease—Greek cosmology wedded to medieval theology. Throughout, she maintains the connection between music and medicine. In fact, she wrote her *Physica* at the same time she composed much of her music.

Healing Harmony in the Later Middle Ages

We have already seen how the pulse was tied to rhythm and harmony and this association continued to be a feature of medical diagnosis throughout the Middle Ages.[77] However, religious music was increasingly the primary form of musical "healing" in the High Middle Ages. Incantations were more religious than magical and limited to the confines of church or prayers by priests offered over the terminally ill. The Church had several rites for the sick or dying. On St. Blaise's day (February 3) it was customary to bless the throats of Roman Catholics in order to prevent diseases of the throats or neck. Blaise was a fourth-century bishop and healer that, legend has it, saved a young girl who was choking on a fish bone.[78] These rituals were usually accompanied by incantations, either sung or spoken. Extreme Unction (The Sacrament of the Sick) is administered when one is dying, though today it is used for anyone who is sick but not necessarily terminal. Incantations are also used when administering the other sacraments. The hymn for the Nativity of St. John the Baptist was sung in the medieval Church to treat the common cold.[79] When Pope Boniface VIII (reigned 1297-1303) was to take a purgative and be phlebotomized, his court musician and poet, Bonaiutus de Casentino, composed two songs for the occasion.[80] The Pope may not have been ill at the time, for in the Middle Ages, it was customary to use purgatives and bloodletting as hygienic measures to maintain good health.

As we have seen, a number of saints were patrons of various aspects of health and sickness. St. Sebastian was the patron saint of those afflicted with or threatened by bubonic plague.[81] Music was composed to accompany prayers to the saint when pestilence threatened a community.[82]

Tarantism

The most curious connection between music and medicine was that found in the disease, "tarantism."[83] It initially occurred in Aquila, a city in the boot of Italy, (sixteenth century) and persisted intermittently for several centuries thereafter. The first scientific studies of Tarantism by physicians were published in the seventeenth century. This disorder was said to be caused by the bite of the Italian tarantula. It was noted that the inhabitants of this dry, hot area of the peninsula were subject to fevers, frenzies, madness, and a host of "inflammatory" diseases. G. Baglivi, a local physician at the time (1723), mentions a high incidence of melancholy in this population. A folk dance, the Tarantella, developed over the years and was said to have resulted from the frenzied dance performed by victims of tarantism. Baglivi asserted that only in Aquila was the tarantula venomous.[84] The "disease" usually occurred in July or August. People would suddenly

jump up with pain after a tarantula bite, although a tarantula was not always seen before the pain began or a bite mark described afterward. The
victim would be compelled to run out of the house and forced to dance
with great excitement. Others who had been bitten in the past, sometimes
several years before, would then join them. It seemed the disease was
never totally cured. Some relapsed annually for as long as thirty years.
Young and old alike were afflicted—one as old as ninety-four. Men and
women were equally prone to the disease. The rich and poor, religious
and secular were similarly victimized. Bright clothes, worn by the danc-
ers, seemed to alleviate the frenzy. Black was abhorrent to the afflicted.
There were those who tore off their clothes and danced nude. Some
howled and made lewd gestures. Others rolled in the dirt and all drank
plentifully of wine. Music and dancing were the only effective remedies.
Deaths were rarely reported. After dancing for several days, the sufferers
would be exhausted and "cured," though playing the Tarantella might
reactivate the frenzied dancing. Over time the disease gradually died out
and patients assumed a normal life After several centuries, the tarantula
bite no longer incited men and women to dance in psychotic frenzies.
There remains, even today, the question whether this was truly a disease
or some form of mass hysteria—possibly a mixture of both.

Gioseffo Zarlino

Gioseffo Zarlino (1517-1590 c.e.) was a deacon at St. Mark's Cathedral
in Venice and acted as music director there, turning down a bishopric in
1583 in order to continue at this famous Byzantine-style church in the
City of Canals. Though he was both a composer and musical theorist,
his *Le Institutioni harmonicho* is considered his most influential work.
Volumes III and IV (1558) deal with counterpoint and modes and are
still read today by musicologists.[85] Just as the number four played a role
in ancient medicine with the humors, qualities and elements, during the
Renaissance this number was important in musical theory.[86] The four
musical elements were the bass, tenor, alto and soprano. The bass was
likened to earth, tenor to water, alto to air and soprano to fire. These four
musical "elements" had the same qualities as the cosmic elements and
played the same role in the musical microcosm as their sublunary coun-
terparts played in the human microcosm. Zarlino notes that composers
most often write four parts that "contain the full perfection of harmony."[87]
Zarlino justifies this analogy as follows:

The movements that give rise to deep sounds are slow and rarified so that by nature...the bass tones are closest to silence. Similarly the earth is by nature immobile
and incapable of sound. The comparison of the treble voice to fire is also justifiable.
High sounds arise from quick frequent movements...and thus participate in the nature
of fire.[88]

Zarlino sees the other two elements and voices as fitting in between earth
and fire. The earth can be most vociferous during earthquakes and fire
often flickers slowly and quietly. Of course, the earth can be very quiet
and fire roar loudly. Zarlino elected to ignore these exceptions since they
were inconsistent with his theoretical construct. At any rate, in music, as
in medicine, Zarlino develops a kind of "humoral" theory. Humors and
qualities determine the nature of music and its effect on the ear. Consonance and dissonance, like health and disease, are determined by these
factors. This theory is extended to the four musical modes in use at the
time: Dorian, Phrygian, Lydian, and Mixolydian. The Dorian mode, for
example, is likened to water and phlegm.

Each mode, according to Zarlino, "was capable of inducing different passions in the souls of the listeners.[89] This may be thought of as
analogous to the four temperaments: phlegmatic, sanguine, cholic, and
melancholic, though he does not ascribe specific modes to each temperament. In fact, he seems to contradict himself at times. For example,
though the Dorian mode is associated with phlegm, suggesting a calm,
impassive personality, he quotes several earlier writers as attributing
severity, bellicosity, majesty or vehemence to this mode. Others say that
virtue, such as chastity, is induced by the Dorian mode. Zarlino believed
the Dorian mode created the most *harmonia* in its hearer, whereas others said that prudence was acquired by listening to this mode. Legend
has it that Agamemnon, before leaving for the Trojan War, left his wife,
Clytemnestra, in the custody of a Dorian musician so that she would
not be corrupted while he was away. The lecherous Aegistus, however,
removed the musician and subsequently had his way with Clytemnestra.
Wisdom was also attributed to this mode. There was little agreement on
the emotional effect of Dorian music.

The Phrygian mode, in contrast, was productive of pleasant, merry
and light moods.[90] It also might be inflammatory, resulting in anger and
wrath, as well as lasciviousness and lust. Similarly, cruelty might be
aroused, according to some writers. Others claimed that madness occurred
in response to Phrygian music. Aristotle called this mode Bacchic—leading to excessive drinking. One philosopher labeled it "religious." Both
Plato and Aristotle prized the Dorian and Phrygian modes, as fostering

wisdom, virtue and citizenship. The Spartans were said to play Phrygian modal music on the trumpet as a call to battle. Certain instruments, such as the trumpet and aulos[91] were judged to favor the Phrygian mode. Zarlino saw the Hypodorian mode as promoting laziness and indolence because of the "heaviness" of its movements. It was, as a consequence, useful in the induction of sleep and relieving the mind of anxiety.

Cassiodorus believed the Lydian mode eased the mind and relaxed the body.[92] Some used this mode in mourning, believing it induced lamentation and weeping. The pipe was best for playing this mode, according to Zarlino. The Hypolydian mode was thought to be full of sweetness—a softer, gentler form of merriment—removing the listener from lasciviousness and every form of vice. It was likened to heavenly happiness. The Mixolydian mode, some believed, might restore sanity.

Zarlino recognizes the variety of effects attributed to each mode and explains these apparent contradictions on changing customs—a warlike society would adopt a mode for this purpose, while peace-loving peoples might use the same mode for its contrary effect. Zarlino also blames these differences on simple ignorance of those writing on the subject. Whatever the utility of the various modes or their effect on the soul and body, it was firmly held that music could impact the harmony of both the *anima* and *corpus*; consequently, music must play an important role in the induction and relief of disease. Conversely, health of both mind and body might be maintained by the use of music in the young, as well as the old.

The application of music in medicine during the Middle Ages and Renaissance was less pervasive than it may have been in Antiquity and the Dark Ages. There certainly was more of a magical, religious aspect to its use in healing. It appears that as healers became more sophisticated, its therapeutic benefit was viewed with increasing skepticism. It was, thus, left to the Church to provide musical healing rather than the physician.

Notes

1. Armstrong, J. 1744, "The Art of Preserving Health" IV, p. 481, This passage has been modified by the author in order to rhyme lines 1 and 2, as well as, lines 3 and 4. These changes are in italics.
2. Radin, P. 1948. *Music and Medicine*, eds. D. M. Schullian and M. Schoen (New York: Henry Schuman), p. 3.
3. Moncrieff, A. R. H. 1992. *A Treasury of Classical Mythology* (New York: Barnes & Noble), p. 9.
4. Hippocrates. 1978. *Hippocratic Writings*, p. 299.
5. The hypotenuse squared (in a right triangle) is equal to the sum of the opposite side squared plus the adjacent side squared: $z^2 = x^2 + y^2$.
6. Radin, 1948. *Music and Medicine*, p. 56.
7. Meinecke, B. 1948, *Music and Medicine*, eds. D. M. Schullian and M. Schoen (New York: Henry Schuman) p. 57.
8. Ibid., p. 58.
9. Ibid., p. 64.
10. Ibid., p. 66.
11. Ibid.
12. Capella, M. 1977. *Martianus Capella*, p. 358.
13. Meinecke, B. 1948. *Music and Medicine* , p. 68.
14. *Anima mundi*: world soul.
15. Meinecke, B. 1948. *Music and Medicine* p. 69.
16. Galen, G. 1997. "The Pulse for Beginners," *Galen: Selected Works*, trans R.N. Singer (New York: Oxford University Press) p. 325.
17. Siraisi, N. G. 1990. *Medieval and Renaissance Medicine*, p. 127.
18. Dactyl: A metrical foot consisting of one accented syllable followed by two unaccented or of one long syllable followed by two short, as in *flattery*. Iamb or iambus: A metrical foot consisting of an unstressed syllable followed by a stressed syllable or a short syllable followed by a long syllable, as in *delay*. In infants, there is often a "split second heart sound" and in adults, the second heart sound is not normally split, i.e., the aortic and pulmonic valves close at the same time. This may be the phenomenon Pietro was referring to. But it is unlikely he listened to the heart. The pulse, at times, may feel as he described it.
19. Guthrie, K. S. 1987. *Pythagorian Source Book*, pp. 24-27.
20. Porphyry, Life of Pythagoras, in Guthrie, K.S. 1987, *Pythagorean Source Book and Library* (Grand Rapids, MI: Phanes Press), p. 129.
21. Plato believed the heavenly bodies to be living divinities as noted above.
22. Guthrie, K.S. 1987. *Pythagorean Source Book*, p. 33.
23. Edelstein, L. 1987, *Ancient Medicine: Selected Papers of Ludwig Edelstein* (Baltimore, MD: Johns Hopkins University Press), pp. 235-237.
24. Hippocrates, vol. II. 1972, p. 147.
25. Veyne, P. 1988, *Did the Greeks Believe in Their Myths?* trans. P. Wissing (Chicago, IL: Chicago University Press), pp. 27-33.
26. Edelstein, L. 1987. *Ancient Medicine*, p. 235.
27. Ibid., Aurelianus, C. *De morbis acutis et chronicus,* 1. c, p. 555.
28. Edelstein, L. 1987. *Ancient Medicine*, p. 236.
29. Ibid. Book I, 179.
30. Op. cit. Hippocrates, vol. II. 1972, p. 147.
31. Galen, *Opera,* ed. Kuhn, XI, p. 792, in Edelstein, L. 1987, p. 237.
32. Ibid., p. 238.
33. Ibid.

34. Ibid., Plato, *Laws*, XI, 935a.
35. Op. cit. Hippocrates, vol. II. 1972, p. 147.
36. Pliny, 1991, *Natural History: A Selection* (New York: Penguin) p. 268.
37. Magic was often practiced in the form of incantations.
38. Ibid., p. 270.
39. Ibid., p. 271.
40. Hippocrates 1972, vol. IV, p. 447.
41. Ibid. p. 346, n. 6
42. Ibid., p. 347.
43. Ibid. p. 348.
44. Ibid., p. 349. Melic verse is intended to be sung.
45. Capella was the first to emphasize the seven Liberal Arts as core subjects for the well-educated academic.
46. Amphion was the son of Zeus and twin brother of Zethus, with whom he built a wall around Thebes by charming the stones into place with the music of his magical lyre.
47. Ibid., p. 352.
48. Ibid., p. 356.
49. Ibid., p. 357.
50. Monad: the Neo-Platonic One or Good, identified with the creator of the Universe.
51. Ibid.
52. Cithara: a stringed instrument similar to a lyre.
53. Asclepiades (124-40 B.C.E.): Physician who established Greek medicine in Rome.
54. Ibid., p. 358.
55. Freeman, C. 2002, *The Closing of the Western Mind: The Rise of Faith and the Fall of Reason* (New York: Vintage/Random House).
56. Boethius, A. 1989, *Fundamentals of Music*, trans. C. M. Bower (New Haven, CT: Yale University Press).
57. Ibid., Book I, 179-180.
58. Lydian and Phrygian modes are ancient keys that were the forerunners of modern day keys such as C major.
59. Op. cit. Plato 1978, p. 115.
60. Chromatic modes are more dissonant and would include modern minor modes such as the key of C minor.
61. Op. cit. Boethius, 1989, Book I, 184.
62. A spondee is a certain poetic rhythm used in ancient songs.
63. Op. cit. Boethius, 1989, Book I, 185.
64. Ibid., Book I, 186.
65. Human music is vocal; instrumental, the music produced by lyre or lute.
66. Ibid., Book I, 188.
67. Ibid.
68 Flanagan, S. 1990, *Hildegard of Bingen, 1098-1179: A Visionary Life* (New York: Routledge) p. 188.
69. Ibid., p. 147.
70. Hildegard claimed to have had visions upon which much of her writings are based. The ideas of winds and airs are echoes of Hippocrates' *Airs, Waters, Places*.
71. Ibid.,
72. Ibid., p. 148.

73. The "nerves" were then thought to function like tendons and ligaments.
74. Op. cit. Flanagan, S. 1990, p. 139.
75. Ibid., p. 140.
76. Op. cit. Siraisi, N. G. 1990, p. 127.
78. Englebert, O. 1994, *The Lives of the Saints*, trans. C. and A. Fremantle (New York: Barnes & Noble) p. 49.
79. Op. cit. Severest, H.E. 1948, p. 96.
80. Ibid., p. 97.
81. Op. cit. Englebert, O. 1994, pp. 26-27.
82. Op. cit. Sierist, H.E. 1948, pp. 99-100.
83. Ibid., pp. 98-114.
84. Tarantula: Any of various large, hairy, chiefly tropical spiders of the family Theraphosidae, capable of inflicting a painful but not seriously poisonous bite. Arizona tarantulas can be generally handled without fear of being bit and even if bitten the wound is usually benign.
85. Zarlino, G. 1968, *De Institutoni Harmoniche*, vol. III, trans. G.A. Marco & C.V. Palisca (New Haven, CT: Yale University Press) and vol. IV, 1983, trans. V. Cohen (New Haven, CT: Yale University Press).
86. Op. cit. Carapetyan, A. 1948, p. 96-122.
87. Op. cit. Zarlino, G. 1968, vol. III, p. 178. Zarlino borrowed this analogy from Luigi Dentice's, *Due dialoghidella musica*, Rome, 1553, second dialogue.
88. Ibid., p. 178.
89. Op. cit. Zarlino, G. 1968, vol. IV, p. 20.
90. Ibid., p. 21.
91. Aulos: a string instrument.
92. Ibid., p. 24.

5

Medieval Medicine in Literature

Geoffrey Chaucer and His Medicine

Geoffrey Chaucer (c.1343-1400) was a man of many talents and interests. He was not formally trained in medicine but was aware of the medical climate of the day. Physicians were not necessarily esteemed by their patients but rather tolerated as the best available medical resource, though not all would agree fully with this judgment. Chaucer's "physik," or physician, as we would call him today, portrays a classic medieval doctor.[1] It is evident from his characterization that Chaucer was well aware of the many aspects of medieval medicine, as well as the professionals who practiced it.

> With us, there was a doctor of physik.
> In all this world ne was there none him like
> To speak of physik and of surgery,
> For he was grounded in astronomy:
> He kept his patïent a full great deal
> In hours, by his magic natural.
> Well could he fórtunen the ascendant
> Of his images for his patient.
> He knew the cause of every malady
> Were it of hot or cold or moist or dry
> And where engendered and of what humor.
> He was a very perfect practiser.
> The cause y-know, and of his harm the root,
> Anon he gave the sickè man his boote.
> His connections with the druggists
> Full ready had he his apothecaries
> To send him drugs and his letuaries,
> For each of them made other for to win;
> Their friendship was not newè to begin.
> Well knew he the old Aesculapius
> And Dioscorides and eke Rusus,

Old Hippocras, Hali and Galen
Serapion, Rasis and Avicen,
Averrois, Damascene and Constantine,
Bernard and Gatesden and Gilbertine.
Of his diet measurable was he *moderate*
For it was of no superfluity *excess*
But of great nourishing and digestible.
His study was but little on the Bible.
In sanguine and in perse he clad was all *In red & blue*
Linèd with taffeta and with sendall, *silk*
And yet he was but easy of dispense. *thrifty spender*
He keptè what he won in pestilence. *during plague*
For gold in physic is a cordial,
Therefore he lovèd gold in specïal.

His portrayal of the medieval "physik" is classic and contains the basic elements of medical theory as has been discussed above.

Chaucer praises the physician's erudite manner and knowledge of medicine. He includes the physik's understanding of surgery, although this is unlikely, since physicians at the time did no surgery and often resisted even touching their patients, preferring to examine the urine and the pulse, leaving surgery to the barber or *chirurgus*.[2] Part of this related to modesty in the case of female patients. All surgery was done by barber-surgeons or "surgeons" who were considered less knowledge-able and who, though a step above the barber-surgeons, were generally not university trained.[3] Astronomy was a major element in medical practice, as noted earlier. The physician was trained in the *Trivium* and *Quadrivium*.[4] The images Chaucer refers to were replicas of the patient or afflicted parts that were hung on the patient at appropriate astrological times with the expectation that the "powers" emanating from celestial objects would enter the patient and provide a kind of healing "magic."[5] Chaucer remarks that the physician knows the cause of every malady. The etiology of disease was based on the ancient Aristotelian-Galenic system of the four humors and four qualities as outlined above. The humors and qualities were, in essence, the same. Phlegm was cold and wet, and an imbalance—excess or deficiency—of one or more of these elements was the root of every illness. Chaucer at this point calls the physician a "very perfect practitioner" who, once arriving at a diagnosis, immediately prescribes the appropriate medicine. The physician had a number of apothecaries who were familiar with the doctor's prescribing patterns and readily made up the required medicines (lectuaries).[6] Chaucer implies that the relationship between the physician and apothecaries is a mutually (monetarily) beneficial arrangement—one not necessarily unethical—but tainted with excessive gain for each.

The physician was well versed in the writings of Asculapius (Asclepius), the legendary son of Apollo (god of medicine) who was so proficient in his profession that he angered the gods by bringing the dead back to life.[7] He is familiar with the writings of Hippocrates, the most famous of ancient physicians.[8] Dioscorides' *Herbal*[9] was the most used such reference.[10] Also mentioned is Galen who was second only to Hippocrates as an influence on medieval medicine. Rusus is likely the Arab physician, Rufus of Ephesus (70-120 C.E.) as was Rasus (al-Razi or Rhazes) (865-925 C.E.). Hali is probably Ali ibn Ridwan (dates unknown), a Cairo astrologer whose writings were translated into English in the twelfth century.[11] Serapion (200-150 B.C.E.) was the founder of the Empirical School of medicine that emphasized observation rather than relying on ancient authorities. Averroes (1126-1198 C.E.) (Ibn Rushd) and Avicenna (discussed previously) were the most famous medieval Arabic doctors. Constantine of Africa a monk at Monte Casino, was the first to translate many Arabic works into Latin.[12] It is unclear who Damascene was. He may have been John Damascene (c. 676-754 C.E.) known primarily as a theologian but also an Aristotelian logician. John of Gaddesden (1280-1349 C.E.), Bernard and Gilbertine compiled medical anthologies (though specifics regarding the last two are lacking).[13]

Chaucer notes that the Physician followed a nourishing, digestible and sparse diet. Diet was a key element in the therapy of medieval medicine and Chaucer makes him out to have practiced what he preached when it came to diet. He was not given to reading the Bible much. This may have been an indication that Chaucer believed most doctors were not very religious. He wore a "blood-red" garment with bluish-grey trim, which was the standard "uniform" (livery) of medieval physicians. They dressed extravagantly so as to set themselves apart from other healers and to emphasize their education and status. It was part of the placebo effect that they relied on so heavily in mediating "cures" since very little of their therapy was truly effective. Chaucer portrays him as parsimonious but having "a special love of gold." In the Middle Ages, many physicians became very wealthy and were often disparaged for their luxurious lifestyle. By the time the Royal College of Physicians was formed in the early sixteenth century,[14] there were only two or three dozen licensed physicians in London and they soon came to monopolize the practice and control of medicine, surgery, and pharmacy.

Chaucer paints a portrait of his physician in a humanistic fashion. The man is not black or white but many shades of gray. In the early Middle Ages, when spirituality was primary, the doctor, priest or politician would have been either a good or evil person. In the time of Chaucer, with humanism creeping into the culture, men and women were being depicted in all aspects of their humanity—a mixture of good and evil—never perfect. A hagiographic picture of any person would no longer work in sculpting a real human being. So it is with Chaucer's Physician. The man he presents has many aspects. Certainly, he was learned for the times. If one reads between the lines, Chaucer seems to suggest that the Physician was not as learned as he would have you believe. Though well read, his reading may not have benefited the patient all that much. It did fill the Physician's purse. One gets the feeling that Chaucer has a sly, sardonic smile on his face as he writes about the Physician—and most of his pilgrims. Indeed, the Physician is much taken with himself—a narcissist in modern psychological parlance. He is more interested in the image he projects than the positive effects of his ministrations. He is a secular man taken with money, having a limited interest in the word of the Bible. He is a businessman more than a practitioner and so it appears are the apothecaries with whom he associates. I think Chaucer's description is an accurate one but he is egalitarian in his depictions—most of the other pilgrims come off looking no better and many much worse.

In outline, Chaucer presents not only the medieval medical man but also the theoretical foundations of medieval medicine. It is all there: the humors, elements, qualities, and their celestial connections, herbal therapy and diet. Though not a compassionate man and taken with money and status, he went about his business, making diagnoses and prescribing therapies.

Notes

1. Chaucer, G.A Middle English version of the *Tales* with modified modernized spelling by Michael Murphy. http://academic.brooklyn.cuny.edu/webcore/murph/canterbury/canterbury.htm. This gives a little flavor of the Middle English in which Chaucer wrote.
2. Chirurgus: Middle English for surgeon.
3. Siraisi, N. G. 1990. Medieval and Renaissance Medicine, pp. 17-48.
4. French, R. 2003. *Medicine Before Science* (Cambridge: Cambridge University Press), p. 77.
5. Chaucer. 1977. *Canterbury Tales*, p. 497.
6. Letuaries, also electuaries: drugs mixed with sugar or honey, made into a pasty mass suitable for oral administration.
7. Edelstein, E.L., and Edelstein, L. 1998. *Asclepius* (Baltimore, MD: Johns Hopkins University Press), p. 56.
8. Hippocrates. 1967 Writings.
9. An herbal a host of medicinal herbs, where they are found, what they look like and the diseases for which they are used.
10. Dioscorides. 1959. *The Greek Herbal of Dioscorides*, ed. R.T. Gunther, (New York: Hafner).
11. O'Neill, Y. V. 1969. "Chaucer and Medicine," *JAMA* 105: 28-82.
12. Ibid.
13. Ibid.
14. Woolley, B. 2004. *Heal Thyself*, p. 34.

Part 3

Moving into Modern Medicine

6

The Faces of Change

From early antiquity, natural philosophers have sought to understand the Universe.[1] How did it begin? Did it have a beginning? What is it composed of and what makes it "tick"? Not surprisingly, the early theories dealt with cosmology and cosmogony. Many of these ancient quests sought to find the elemental basis for our world. Thales (c. 624-c.546 B.C.E.) proposed water as the single material cause of all earthly things.[2] Subsequently, Anaximander (611-547 B.C.E.) offered a totally different primordial element as the "stuff" of which all things are made, namely, the Infinite or απειρον (apeiron). [3] This was a metaphysical concept that, to this day, is not well understood. The apeiron or eternal, indeterminate, infinite substance was a metaphysical monadic material capable of separating into opposites, such as heavy and light, hot and cold and so on from whence all things emanate.[4] Anaximenes (c. 545 B.C.E.) suggested air as the one, infinite cause of the physical world. Heraclitus (c. 500 B.C.E.) maintained that fire was the prime element, emphasizing change as the one vital force in the Universe; this best fit his model of conflict and change essential to Nature.[5] Empedocles is generally given credit for adding earth to the other three elements, fire, air, and water, thus rounding out a theory of "sublunary" cosmology.[6] The Ancients believed that the sublunary world—the Earth and its surrounding air—was made of these four elements, was always in a state of flux and all motion on Earth was "rectilinear," that is, in a straight line. The Moon and all celestial objects beyond it were made of "ether" and moved in circles. Ether, unlike the four earthly elements, was immutable and eternal. We have already been introduced to these early philosophical concepts.

Because many ancient physicians were also astronomers, these four elements came to play an important role in their theory of medicine. We have seen Pythagoras' dual role as astronomer and healer.[7] Eudoxus, who was the first to posit concentric orbits for the Sun, Moon and five planets as they moved around the Earth, was a practicing physician[8] as was Empedocles.[9] It is understandable that these astronomer-physicians would be inclined to use cosmology in their attempt to understand the medicine they practiced. As we have also seen, this tradition was adopted by Hippocrates, Aristotle, and Galen and provided the bases for medical theory and practice for the next two millennia. This theoretical structure of medicine, however, began to crumble in the sixteenth century with the emerging Enlightenment. Copernicus, a Catholic cleric, physician, and astronomer, dealt the first blow to the theory of ancient and medieval medicine. He was followed in the destruction and reconstruction of medical theory by Vesalius, the anatomist, Galileo, Newton, and others, all of whom added another nail to the coffin of early medical theory and practice. This section will catalogue these and other men and the ideas they brought to Western Europe during the post-Renaissance period. Elizabethan practitioners, who represent the transitional phase from old to new medicine, will be discussed followed by the medical changes of the eighteenth century.

Roger Bacon Begins the End

Roger Bacon (c.1214-c.1292 C.E.) was a man of manifold mysteries.[10] His birth date and many facets of his career are obscured by the fog of history. It is known that Roger Bacon was one of the first true experimental scientists—a man centuries ahead of his time. As is often the case with such men of genius, especially if they are intolerant of their superiors and freely critical of their fellow academics, trouble is sure to follow on their heels like the Hound of Heaven. But in spite of Bacon's many failings, he was not only a learned student of practical science but a holistic thinker who brought together many disciplines to form a unified vision of the world in a way not previously imagined.

Roger Bacon's Life

Roger Bacon was born in the second decade of the thirteenth century near Ilchester, Somersetshire, England.[11] He came into an affluent farming family but because he was not the eldest son, it was expected that he would pursue some career other than agriculture. Oxford, at the time, was in its infancy. The University had been granted a royal charter in 1214 and Roger, who at age thirteen had most likely never been outside Somerset, made the journey east to the little town of Oxford to begin a career in academics. Undoubtedly, he had studied Latin grammar, the elements of rhetoric and Aristotelian logic (the *Trivium*) locally before matriculating at Oxford. The University, at the time, was a series of "houses" where the students lived and studied under a Master who held a degree equivalent to our current M.A. This Master's degree followed four years of arithmetic, astronomy, geometry and music (the *Quadrivium*). Two more years were then devoted to theology, philosophy, law, or medicine. This was the road followed by Bacon. Natural philosophy, that is, "science," was of most interest to him. He never became a "Doctor"; this would have required as much as sixteen additional years of study, teaching and writing. After teaching at Oxford for a time, possibly five or six years, he crossed the channel to take a post at the University of Paris around 1242 where he stayed for another five or six years. He was an Aristotelian through and through. Bacon viewed speculative philosophy, of the sort advocated by Plato, as inferior to the more hands-on science of Aristotle. One of Roger's pet peeves focused on academics who sat at their desks pondering the Ancients and writing commentaries about their works, using "reason" as the only measure of truth. Aristotle had not been well received in Paris because of his teachings concerning the eternity of the world—a view contrary to Catholic doctrine and at odds with Genesis.[12] As a result, there were few who could teach Aristotle at Paris and Bacon was brought there, in part, to fill this academic void.

At Paris, he was influenced in a major way by Petrus Peregrinus de Maricourt. Petrus Peregrinus was an experimental scientist and though only one of his works, *De magnete* (On magnets), survives, it is evident from this work and what Bacon says of him in the *Opus majus* (his best known and largest work) that Petrus was a hands-on scientist and influenced Bacon in his later research. Following a suppression of Aristotelian doctrines at Paris, Bacon returned to Oxford around 1250. This move was prompted not only by the University's rejection of Aristotle but also by Bacon's desire to join like-minded colleagues and possibly find a more stable situation academically and financially.

Bacon entered the Franciscan Order in the 1250s, possibly as late as 1257. Roger Bacon was an independent thinker with a penchant for arousing the ire of his peers. He certainly was not one to acquiesce to the opinions of others; so the reasons for his decision to join a mendicant order with a rigid hierarchy, where he was bound not only by poverty and chastity, but also by unquestioning obedience to his superiors, is a puzzle. He may have naively believed that he could overcome all these limitations by the sheer force of his intellect. This never happened and

Roger spent some time in both Paris and Oxford under a *de facto* "house arrest" imposed by his superiors for opposing "modernization" of the order and many of his writings, which did not meet with the approval of the Church hierarchy.

In 1266, Bacon, who had made the acquaintance of a certain Cardinal Guy de Foulques, later Pope Clement IV, wrote the new Pope about his research and Clement asked Roger to send him an example of his work. Bacon composed feverishly for a full year. The product was the *Opus majus*, his masterpiece. The tome was delivered to Clement but shortly after this, on November 29, 1268, Clement died plunging Bacon into deep despair.

Some time following this, Bacon returned to England and tradition has it that he became increasingly critical of his fellow professors, including Albertus Magnus (c.1206-1280) who was a well thought of academic. Whatever the reasons, it appears that Roger Bacon spent the last ten or fifteen years of his life in solitary confinement in a friary near Oxford. Bacon lived in squalid conditions, unable to continue his writing, deprived of friends, given minimal food and water, and denied the Sacraments, thus, condemned to eternal damnation, according to Church doctrine.[13] Bacon never truly recanted any of the "novelties," that is, heterodoxy, he was accused of, but it is said that on his death-bed he moaned, "I repent of having given myself so much trouble in destroying ignorance!"

The Science of Roger Bacon

Roger Bacon states unequivocally that, "without experiment it is impossible to know anything thoroughly."[14] He maintains that the principles of wisdom are found in experimental science. Bacon asserts there are two ways of acquiring knowledge—reason and experiment.[15] There is certitude in mathematics but reason can only take the philosopher so far. Certitude in the world comes only from experimental science. Reasoning without experience can be "wholly false."[16] Essential to true wisdom is knowledge of causes and these can be ascertained with certainty only through experiments. Bacon is highly critical of "Doctors of Theology" such as Albertus Magnus and Thomas Aquinas who entered religious life at a young age and studied philosophy and theology without ever seeing the world through the prism of experimental science. He supported Aristotle, who under Alexander the Great, sent out 2,000 men to gather experimental data.[17] Speculative "science" is prone to error. He notes errors in Pliny's *Natural History* based on "facts" that have not been tested by experiment. As an example, he pooh poohs Pliny's contention that adamant[18] can only be broken by the blood of a goat. Philosophers and theologians had perpetuated this myth having never tested its truth or falsity. Bacon goes on to say that this claim about adamant is not true; that it can be broken by other means and that he has seen it done. He says, "I have seen this with my eyes," thus affirming the validity of the senses in the acquisition of knowledge. Sense knowledge had not always been accepted as a valid measure of truth.

Bacon goes on to claim that experience (experimental science) can be obtained in two ways:

> One is through the external senses such are the experiments that are made upon the heavens through instruments in regard to facts there, and (secondly) the facts on earth that we prove in various ways to be certain in our own sight.[19]

What he is referring to when speaking of "instruments" used to acquire facts about heaven is uncertain though he does predict the invention of the telescope.[20] The astrolabe had been available since the first century B.C.E. and used by both astronomers and navigators. Various "line of sight" methods were then used for observing the stars before 1609 when Galileo first constructed his telescope. Bacon experimented with lenses and mirrors as well as alchemy and was familiar with the methods employed in optics and chemistry and other earthly sciences.

Bacon does admit the utility of reason in the form of logic and states that though the facts need to be acquired experimentally, logic is necessary to provide correct conclusions. He says, "Scientists know that their principles come from experiment but the conclusions through…this noble science (logic)." In other words, sense gives data, logic provides the proper interpretation of these data.

Bacon's most extensive and thorough studies concerned optics. Light had held a place in Christian thought for centuries and Robert Grosseteste (1168-1253 C.E.), one of Bacon's mentors, had written a quasi-scientific treatise on light.[21] Whatever Bacon's stimulus, he spent a great deal of time experimenting on light using mirrors and lenses.[22] He found this work "far nobler and more pleasing" than even the study of mathematics. Bacon believed, along with the Ancients, that vision was the result of a beam of light emanating from the eye itself, which radiated into space to connect with some light from the object seen. From this union vision resulted. This was purely speculative theory based on his reading of other authors. But he did accomplish some true science in his study of light.

Bacon describes the anatomy of the brain. He correctly associated the eyes with the optic nerves that, in turn, connect the eyes to the brain. He was aware of the optic chiasm, where the optic nerves cross before entering the brain proper. Bacon may not have actually dissected the brain but rather drew from the work of others; however, he did interpret the data properly. He also describes the anatomy of the eye in some detail. He did do hands-on experiments with lenses and mirrors, laying out the optics of reflection and refraction. Bacon's most extensive work on light was *De multiplicatione specierum* but this was an entirely speculative work.

As noted above, Bacon believed:

> We may read the smallest letters at an incredible distance, we may see object however small they may be, and we may cause the stars to appear wherever we wish.[23]

All this was to be done using lenses, according to Bacon. That Bacon ever attempted to carry out these studies is doubtful but he did understand the concepts behind such devices as telescopes and microscopes. It wasn't until 300 years later that the father and son team of Leonard and Thomas Digges[24] first assembled a working telescope and some time later that Hans and Zacharias Janssen constructed a microscope—the one revolutionizing astronomy, the other biology,[25] that Bacon's predictions came to pass.

Roger Bacon was fascinated by alchemy. He experimented with the explosive power of gunpowder. He failed, however, to understand the propulsive force of this substance.

In his letter *De mirabile potestate artis et natura* (On the marvelous power of art and nature), Bacon sets out a list of wonders that would not come to fruition for several centuries. He envisioned seagoing vessels powered by means other than sails or oarsmen that could be handled by but one person. He also imagined a "car" that would move with "inestimable speed" using no "living creature" to move it. He believed there would be "flying machines." Not an entirely new concept as the myth of Icarus reminds us. It is of interest that Bacon claims to have seen all of the inventions he wrote about except the "flying machine." Many of these inventions, he falsely believed, had been used earlier by the Ancients. He understood the enormous potential of pulley systems and imagined them being put to tasks of great magnitude, never before accomplished. He suggested such a system could allow many men to escape from prison at one time or as a means of dragging a thousand men, during battle, close enough to easily destroy them. Bacon envisioned an invention that would allow a man to walk on the bottom of the sea. There is no evidence that Bacon or his mentor Petrus Peregrinus actually constructed any of these contraptions. It is certain that Bacon spent a great deal of money on his research (and buying books), so that he must have been very actively experimenting, especially before he entered the Franciscan Order. Whether there were specific projects that he described and which have since been lost is unknown. Legend has it that after his death, much of his work was burned by the Oxford friars but this is conjectural and may have related to the myth of Roger Bacon that arose in the centuries after his death.

While Bacon was in a friary near Paris, possibly for reasons of health, he worked on updating the calendar. Since Julius Caesar's reform of the calendar in 46 B.C.E. the calendar had gotten out of step with the stars and Sun. The equinoxes (when the Sun appears to cross the Earth's equator) were off by seven days or so by the thirteenth century. Bacon realized this missed timing was important for several reasons. Planting of crops could be affected as well as the date for Easter. The *Computus* was the procedure used to set the time of Easter during the Middle Ages and it was considered the most important ecclesiastical and astronomical calculation of the Church year. Bacon corrected the calendar and even wrote the Pope suggesting that he implement the change. Nothing was done until Pope Gregory XIII made the appropriate changes in 1582.

Another contribution Bacon made to the modern world concerns Christopher Columbus. In his *Opus majus*, he suggests that it should be possible to head west from Spain and arrive at India.[26] This section of the *Opus* was taken almost verbatim by Cardinal Pierre d'Ailly and incorporated into his *Imago mundi* that was one of the sources Columbus used in planning his voyage to the New World!

It is evident that Roger Bacon was a man ahead of his time; unfortunately, as noted earlier, he fell afoul of medieval conservatives—so long wedded to ancient authority. It is not that he held heretical views—divine inspiration was, in his mind, more certain than experimentation. But he ran counter to modernizing trends taking place in the Franciscan Order and undoubtedly ruffled hierarchical feathers, which ultimately led to his downfall.

Bacon and his works were little read after his death. In subsequent centuries, a mystique developed around his life and works. In time, books and plays appeared fictionalizing his life. In the Victorian period, English translations of his writings became available and he was transformed into a popular national figure. The Victorians even claimed him as one of their own. All of the facts of his life may never be known but recent scholarship has begun to unearth more about the "real" Roger Bacon and this work allows us to define his place in the history of science, so that he may be given the credit due him as a scientific thinker. He was, unquestionably, one of the very earliest "true" scientists.

Leonardo da Vinci

Leonardo da Vinci (1452-1519) was born 15 April 1452 in the small Tuscan town of Vinci.[27] His father, Piero da Vinci, was a notary and his mother, Caterina, was most likely a peasant girl. Piero married another woman the sixteen-year-old Albiera Amadori, later that year. Because Leonardo was illegitimate, he did not receive the education afforded most sons of a notary. Consequently, he was largely self-taught.

Giorgio Vasari (1511-1574), a painter and the designer of the Uffizi in Florence and biographer of many Renaissance artists, says of Leonardo:

> Celestial influences may shower extraordinary gifts on certain human beings, which is an effect of nature; but there is something supernatural in the accumulation in one individual of so much beauty, grace and might.[28]

Not only did Leonardo possess grace and good looks, he was said to be strong enough to bend a horseshoe with his bare hands. It is thought that Raphael used him as the model for Plato in *The School of Athens.*

In this picture, Raphael not only portrays Leonardo but also defines both the distinction and unity of the heavens and earth, reinforcing the connection between the harmony of heaven and that of human health.

Leonardo da Vinci was the ultimate polymath: painter, musician, architect, and engineer. He worked with a variety of media, oils on wood (the *Mona Lisa*), tempera, chalk and cast bonze among others. He orchestrated gala festivals, and played the *lira da braccio,* a forerunner of the viola. He was so proficient with this instrument that when introduced at the Milanese court, it was as a musician and not as a painter.[29] His interests were wide-ranging: geology,[30] optics, acoustics, mathematics, military machines, urban planning, hydraulics, ballistics, botany, and health, to mention a few. His mind moved at such a pace that he failed to complete many of his projects. There are fewer than twenty paintings attributed to him, though hundreds of drawings remain. These sketches were often the preliminary musings of the artist or the result of rambling ideas emanating from his imagination that then flowed onto a sketchpad.

For our present purposes, it is his anatomy, physiology, and harmonic theory that are of interest. Leonardo da Vinci was neither physician nor apothecary but in his many notebooks there are numerous references and drawings devoted to such topics. It is in his notes that we find his medical and paramedical ruminations.

Leonardo's Anatomy

Da Vinci's anatomy flowed from his artistic interests. Nicoll asserts that his anatomical drawings represent a totally new way of portraying the human body.[31] This may, indeed, be the case, for his humanism and realism combined to create the most remarkable anatomical depictions yet devised —to be surpassed only by Vesalius less than fifty years later.[32] There had been an implicit, if not explicit, ecclesiastical prohibition against human dissection during the Middle Ages.[33] Whatever the Church's official position, there was a negative view of autopsies during this period. Anatomy was based on Galenic principles and, thus, derived from animal studies. The first openly performed autopsy was in 1286.[34] This was done in order to ascertain the cause of death in a plague victim. By 1302, autopsies were often performed in Bologna in suspected criminal cases. In 1316, Mundinius (c. 1270-1326) published the *Anothomia*, which was the first book of its kind devoted entirely to anatomy and physiology. It was based largely on human dissections performed by Mundinius himself. Up to this time, anatomical illustrations had been limited to the so-called "Five Picture Series." This genre, derived from Egyptian and Greek sources, consisted of five views of the human body showing the bones, muscles, nerves, veins, and arteries in a semi-squatting figure. A sixth figure was added later depicting a pregnant woman or the male or female genital anatomy. These were rigid, stylized figures. Dissection was officially sanctioned by the University of Bologna in 1405.

Giotto di Bondone (1267-1337) is generally considered the first "naturalistic" painter of the early Renaissance. Undoubtedly, Leonardo was influenced by Giotto as the humanistic movement began to flower.

Andrea del Verrocchio (1435-1488), Leonardo's tutor, followed in the mold of Giotto and further influenced da Vinci's artistic realism. Nonetheless, he was a scientist at heart and this penchant for the earthly world below rather than the spiritual one above, drove him to seek first hand knowledge in all his endeavors. He dissected more than thirty cadavers—mostly male and female criminals—which provided the models for his drawings.[35] Leonardo was left-handed and could write backwards from right to left, reversing not only words but letters as well—to be read with a mirror. It has been suggested that he did so in order to conceal some of his necropsy descriptions, too discreditable to preserve his reputation.

Leonardo covers the skeletal, muscular, cardiovascular, digestive and genitourinary systems in his anatomy drawings. See figure 6.1. His depictions though realistic, are not as humanistic as Vesalius' representations are, as is evident below. These drawings are more accurately done than in the past but don't achieve the "living" anatomy of Vesalius.

In addition to his anatomical work, Leonardo shows an interest in and knowledge of physiology. In 1489, he completed eight studies of the human skull. One of these deals with intracranial nerves and blood vessels. Da Vinci attempts to explain the psychology of sensation or the *sensus communis* postulated by Aristotle.[36] Following dissections of the head done in 1489, Leonardo writes in his notebook:

> Where the line a-m is intersected by the line c-b, there will be the confluence of all the senses.

He is trying to localize the *sensus communis*, the part of the brain where sensory impressions are coordinated and interpreted. This area was one of three important brain centers, the other two the *impresiva*, where sensory input is gathered and the memoria, a storage site for processed information (memory). The *sensus communis* is the center of judgment and the location of the soul.[37] This is a highly speculative scheme and bears the marks of metaphysical philosophy rather than true neurophysiology. Da Vinci's efforts in other areas of anatomy and physiology are less speculative, at times based on human dissections but always on Galenic principles established centuries before. An example of this is found in his studies of the cardiovascular system. Along with other writers of the Middle Ages and early Renaissance, da Vinci believed that blood did not circulate but swished back and forth within the arteries and veins. Blood was produced in the liver from ingested nutrients. This was a continual process, necessary because circulation of blood had not yet been discovered by William Harvey. All blood was believed to be used up when it reached the various bodily tissues. It was estimated by da Vinci that seven ounces of blood was consumed hourly.[38] Since blood was manufactured from ingested food stuffs, it was easy for da Vinci to accept the humoral theory of health and disease. If unhealthy

Figure 6.1
Examples of da Vinci's Musculoskeletal Drawings

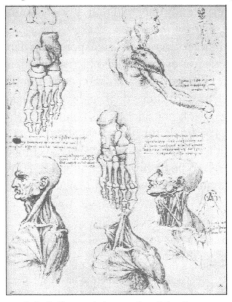

foods were ingested, it followed that unhealthy humors and consequent disease would follow.

Leonardo's anatomy of the heart was largely derived from dissection of the ox heart.[39] His cardiovascular physiology followed Galen with modifications. Much of his work was taken from Mundinius' *Anothomia,* which, as noted, was the first medieval attempt to depict human anatomy based on cadaver dissections. Using these sources, da Vinci believed the blood, after leaving the liver, traveled via the inferior vena cava to the right "auricle" or atrium as it is usually labeled today.[40] From this chamber of the heart, it was pumped into the right ventricle. This occurred during ventricular diastole (when the ventricle was not contracting) allowing the blood to flow unimpeded from the auricle to the ventricle. During ventricular systole, the blood went in three directions. It refluxed into the right auricle through the open tricuspid valve, into the pulmonary artery and thence to the lungs and, finally, through the interventricular septal "pores" leading to the left ventricle. Within the left ventricle, "vital heat" was added to the blood and then transferred to the rest of the body. Also, pneuma from the lungs passing along the pulmonary vein cooled the blood in the left ventricle. If the body became overheated, breathing faster brought more air into the blood, thus cooling it and reducing disease causing heat. As we have seen, if the blood was too hot, disease resulted as well. The flux and reflux of the blood into the right auricle and in and out of the aorta "subtlized" the blood making it (through friction) hot and thin; it was therefore more healthy, according to Galenists of the time.

The existence of interventricular septal pores was debated for centuries and, of course, none was ever identified.[41] There were many inconsistencies and errors in Leonardo's anatomical and physiological concepts of the muscular, skeletal, gastrointestinal, and genitourinary systems. These errors are understandable considering his failure to perform physiological studies, his use of animals for dissection and the prevailing "wisdom" of the age. Aristotle and Galen still held sway over medical practice and theory and were not to be dethroned for another 150 years.

Leonardo reiterates many aspects of Galen and other ancients when he asserts that:

> Man has been called by the ancients a lesser world and indeed the term is rightly applied, seeing that if man is compounded of earth, water, air and fire this body of the earth is the same. As man has within himself bones as a stay and framework for the flesh, so the world has the rocks which are the supports of the earth. As man has within him a pool of blood wherein the lungs as he breathes expand and contract, so the body of the earth has its ocean, which also rises and falls every six hours with the breathing of the world.[42]

He goes on to compare the veins of man with the rivers of Earth. Once again, we see the four elements and man as the microcosm, though in this instance it is the Earth that is the macrocosm. He also claims that the Sun gives spirit and life to the plants. And though he discusses botany at length, it is more with the eye of the artist than that of the healer or philosopher. He speaks of the Earth as a living being. It has a spirit of growth. And it possesses, like the human body, its flesh, which is the soil. [43] The rocks are its bones, its cartilage the tufa[44] and its blood as mountain springs of water. These springs he likens to a boil that pours out pus, thus cleansing the earth. [45] Water rises to a mountain top just as blood flows to the head. And as the springs are warmed by summer sunshine the vital heat warms the blood of humans. Leonardo obviously sees man, the microcosm, as having much in common with Earth, the mcrocosm.

In terms of harmony, we hear da Vinci echo ancient voices. As noted earlier, he was a skilled musician and harmony was ever present in all his works, whether painting, building or performing. The most famous of his connections between humans and harmony is in the "Vitruvian Man," named after the famous first-century Roman architect, Vitruvius, it

Figure 6.2
The Vitruvian Man

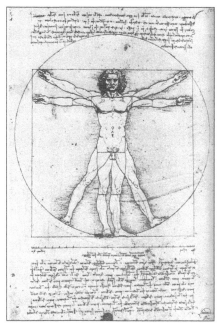

purports to show the divine harmony of human anatomy— the mathematical ratios of the body. Vitruvius was the first to lay out the classical theory of human harmonious proportions.[46] Leonardo did a number of sketches on this topic, many in the Royal Library at Windsor and several others that are lost and known to us only through copies. The most famous, of these is shown in figure 6.2. also known as the *Homo ad circulum*, currently in the Academia of Venice. Leonardo explains the human body in terms of ratios of one part of the body to other parts. In the notes accompanying the drawing, Leonardo enumerates these ratios:

> The measurements of man are distributed by Nature as follows: that 4 fingers make one palm, and 4 palms make one foot; 6 palms make one cubit [a forearm, from the Latin cubitus, elbow], 4 cubits make a man's height. And 4 cubits make one pace and 24 palms make a man.[47]

He goes on to further define the harmony of the body:

> Hairline to chin = 1/10th a man's height.
> Top of head to chin = 1/8th "   "
> Top of head to breast = 1/8th "   "
> Roots of hair to breasts = 1/7th   "
> Top of head to nipple = 1/4th   "
> Width of the shoulders = 1/4th   "

Elbow to tip of hand = 1/5th   "
Elbow to armpit [axilla[= 1/8th   "
Whole hand = 1/10th   "
The genitals mark the middle of a man
Foot = 1/7th part of a man.
etc. [48]

The Vitruvian Man is enclosed in both a square and a circle. The square measures 96 fingers (24 palms). The center of the outstretched limbs is the umbilicus (navel) and the legs form an equilateral triangle. The center of the circle is the umbilicus. The outstretched arms perpendicular to the torso are equal in length to the height of the man. This figure, obviously, is filled with harmonic ratios in the manner of Pythagoras. However, da Vinci expresses in the Vitruvian Man both harmony and humanism, two hallmarks of the Renaissance. In this figure, he echoes the harmony of heaven as found in humans and first elaborated by the Ancients centuries before. Leonardo takes several steps forward, however, in this portrayal of the human figure. It is no longer a stylized medieval man. This man prefigures the Vesalius man of 1543. Though Leonardo was undoubtedly one of the world's great artists, his representations of the human anatomy fall far short of the work by Vesalius. Nonetheless, Leonardo has to be counted among the giants upon whose shoulders modern medicine was built. In spite of all his efforts, many errors are found in his sketches that can be blamed on his limited access to human material, the elementary understanding of medicine at the time and the primary purpose for his anatomical sketches—to provide artists with a proper approach to depicting the human body. Whether Vesalius used or was influenced by da Vinci is unknown. Nonetheless, Leonardo was part of the revolution taking place during the Renaissance that ultimately made way for the Enlightenment. It is very likely that Leonardo influenced Vesalius either directly or indirectly, if not by his anatomical artistry, at least by his humanism.

Nicolas Copernicus

Nicolas Copernicus (1473-1543 C.E.) was a canon[49] at the cathedral in Frombork (in present-day Poland). He was also a university trained physician who practiced medicine most of his life. It was not, however, as a physician that Copernicus impacted the future course of medicine. Rather, it was his work in astronomy that provided one of the first blows to the theory of medieval medicine.[50] In his most famous work, *De Revolutionibus*, he lays out the mathematical basis for the heliocentric theory of the Solar System.[51] For centuries, the Bible had been interpreted as describing a geocentric world with the immobile Earth at its center; the Moon, Sun, planets, and stars all revolving around God's most important creation. It was not only a geocentric but also an egocentric system. Humans were the highest creatures God had made—they were special and the Universe was considered to have been created for us humans who were "rational animals" and, as such, reigned above all other creatures, excepting the angels. If the Earth was *not* at the center of the Universe, then how could we mortal beings be at the center of God's creative plan? If Copernicus' paradigm was correct, we would no longer be as special as once thought. This was not only a crippling blow to our ego but brought into question the whole of the Bible—the very heart of Western religion. Even more disturbing was the damage this could do to Aristotle, who was a geocentrist and the most esteemed natural philosopher of the ancient and medieval worlds. If Aristotle was wrong, so was Galen, upon whose authority (along with Hippocrates) rested all medical theories of the day. If Galen was wrong, then physicians had been doing medicine all wrong for nearly 2,000 years!

Copernicus knew the distress his theory would bring to the Church.

> Since the newness of the hypotheses of this work—which sets the Earth in motion and puts an immovable Sun at the center of the Universe…I have no doubt that certain of the savants have taken grave offense and think it wrong to raise any disturbance among liberal disciplines which have had the right set up for a long time now. [52]

It was only with great reluctance that he was induced to publish *De Revolutionibus* a few months before his death—dedicating it to Pope Paul III as a peace offering to the Church.

Copernicus' system was presented only as a theory to explain observed celestial motions. Ptolemy (c. 109-175 c.e.) had developed a system that provided reasonably good predictability of stellar and planetary positions but it involved a number of "fudge factors" such as epicycles and equants (see appendix) made necessary because the Earth wasn't actually at the center of the Solar System and the Moon and planets did not follow perfectly circular orbits rather, elliptical ones.[53]

Copernicus, as a skilled mathematician, knew that Ptolemy's approach was imperfect:

> We see that very many things (celestial positions) are not in accord with the movements which should follow from his (Ptolemy's) doctrine.…Whence even Plutarch

in speaking of the revolving solar year says, "so far the movement of the stars has overcome the ingenuity of the mathematicians."[54]

Copernicus was not the first to question the geocentric system,[55] but he did not abandon Ptolemy entirely. He maintained, in true Aristotelian fashion, that all celestial bodies move in perfect circular orbits—including the Earth.[56] In order to account for the discrepancies noted in Ptolemy's scheme, he included epicycles but not equants. It is of interest that using this modified geometry, the actual path planets followed was in reality elliptical, although the defererns and epicycles were still perfect circles. Even with these adjustments, Copernicus' approach fails to perfectly predict the course of the planets. It was Kepler who was to explain these discrepancies sixty years later using elliptical orbits for the planets.

One would think that earlier astronomers might have tumbled to the fact that celestial orbits were elliptical and not circular, but divine, super-lunary bodies demanded (in the minds of philosophers such as Aristotle) the mathematically perfect circle for their orbits. This was typical of the speculative reasoning that permeated the ancient and medieval mind. Besides, Aristotle was *the* Philosopher and could not be wrong. Such authorities were sacrosanct during the Middle Ages and questioning their credibility was considered virtual heresy at the time. Men were burned at the stake for such beliefs.

In time, Copernicus' system caught the eye of such noted astronomers as Galileo Galilei and Johannes Kepler but it took more than two centuries for it to be generally accepted by the academic world.

Tycho Brahe

The next several blows dealt to medieval medical theory also came from astronomers. One night in 1572, Tycho Brahe (1546-1601 c.e.), while at Herrevad Abbey developing technical instrumentation, looked up at the sky and noticed an object he had never seen before.[57] It was a supernova—an aging star that had exploded in some distant part of our Milky Way Galaxy.[58] He followed the brightness of this "new star" until it faded into nothingness months later. These observations were published in *De mundi atherei recentioribus phanomenis*, which was intended to be the first of a five-volume set attacking the cosmology of Aristotle, who had held that, as divine, perfect beings, stars were eternally immutable. They neither wander about the sky, as is the case with the Moon, Sun, and planets, nor change their luminosity. Here was clear evidence that Aristotle was wrong. If "The Philosopher" could be in error with regard to the stars, he might also be wrong with regard to the workings of the human body.

A supernova had been reported in China and Japan in 1181 C.E.[59] but apparently went unnoticed in the Western World. By chance, another supernova appeared in 1604 and almost two centuries later, the first Cepheid variable was observed by John Goodwicke in 1784.[60] Cepheids, it turns out, vary in brightness over a period of days to weeks and these "variable" stars provided additional evidence that stars were neither "fixed" nor immutable further weakening this ancient, time honored belief.

Johannes Kepler

Ancient medical theory was further weakened by the work of Brahe's pupil, Johannes Kepler (1571-1630 C.E.). Although Brahe died two years after Kepler joined him, his astrometric data[61] were so accurate that they allowed Kepler to develop his three famous laws. The first law states that planets (and other objects such as comets) move in elliptical orbits, contradicting the Ancients' dictum that superlunary bodies followed perfect circular orbits. In addition, Kepler demonstrated, in his second law that planets moved faster when nearer the Sun.[62] This was another inconsistency in Aristotle's scheme, since superlunary objects were supposed to move at a constant velocity at all times. This was part of their assumed divine immutability. Using Brahe's data, Kepler was able to prove that celestial bodies did not follow the dicta laid down by the Ancients. Could the stars and planets be less than divine beings and more like our Earth?

Galileo Galilei

In 1610, Galileo (1564-1642 C.E,) using a telescope he had constructed following the lead of Dutch lens-makers, discovered the four innermost moons of Jupiter.[62] This discovery created a furor in Western Europe, involving both cosmology and religion. Now there were eleven satellites, instead of the time-honored seven, which disturbed the religious magic of the number seven discussed previosly. This number was considered sacred. There were seven capital sins and virtues, fourteen Stations of the Cross (seven on either side of church), seven days of the week, the early rosary had seven "decades" and seven is considered a lucky number, even today. There were seven metals known at the time and each had been assigned to a planet—lead to Saturn, tin to Jupiter, etc. More importantly, these four Jovian satellites were revolving around Jupiter and not Earth.

Earth was no longer the center of the Universe as Aristotle and many others had proclaimed for so many centuries. Further, Galileo observed that the Moon was not "perfect"—it possessed mountains and valleys with many irregular surface features—making it no longer a perfect, ethereal sphere; it looked a lot like our own planet. Earth was supposed to be the only imperfect, mutable creation of God. In this same vein, Galileo saw that the Sun had sunspots—features that had been observed for many centuries, but now the telescope verified that the Sun was "mutable" as well—this was neither compatible with the cosmology of Aristotle nor the theology of medieval churchmen. Finally, Galileo observed the phases of Venus—evidence that this planet revolved around the Sun and not Earth. This was not as devastating as the other findings of Galileo, for Tycho Brahe had earlier devised a compromise system that included both geocentric and heliocentric features in order to preserve the primacy of Earth. Added to all this "new astronomy" was the observation of another supernova by Galileo in 1604, mentioned earlier.[63]

René Descartes: His Life

René Descartes (1596-1650) was born 31 March 1596 in the small village of La Haye near Chatellerault in the region of Tourraine.[64] Joachim Descartes, René's father, was a lawyer. His maternal great-grandfather, Jean Ferrand, was a physician. Jean's daughter, Claude, married Pierre Descartes, also a physician, and René's paternal grandfather. Pierre died young of urinary stones. His father-in-law is said to have performed his autopsy, following which he published a treatise on renal lithiasis (kidney stones), *Traité des maladies de la pierée.*

Joachim Descartes married Jeanne Brochard. They had three children, Pierre, Jeanne and René. Their mother died the next year of tuberculosis when René was only 13 months old. René later believed he inherited a pale color and chronic, dry cough from his mother and was told by local physicians that he would not survive till adulthood. His father remarried and moved to Rennes, leaving Jeanne and René to be cared for by their maternal grandmother. At age ten, René entered the Jesuit College at La Fleche. Etienne Charlet, a relative of René, was rector at the College. Whether it was Fr. Charlet s influence, René was a "favored" student and allowed to sleep late and study in his room—a habit he maintained the rest of his life. Though weak appearing, René became a horseman, learned fencing, which he dearly loved, and played skittles (a form of bowling).

The study of religion, philosophy, and science, along with languages, history, oratory, and poetry, filled his academic life. As was the tradition at the time, the Jesuits taught the philosophy of Aristotle and Thomas Aquinas. Descartes was later to renounce Scholastic philosophy in favor of a more "modern" system based on the dualism of mind-body and a mechanical view of the physical world. These two concepts play a major role in his theory of medicine.

Descartes is considered by many to be the first "modern" philosopher. This, along with a "scientific" mind-set, makes him a person to be included among those who shaped Enlightenment medicine. He was first and foremost a keen mathematician, credited with developing analytical geometry. It was the demonstrative aspect of mathematics that he used in structuring his philosophical proofs of being and the existence of God.

In 1614, René matriculated in the Faculty of Law at Poitiers, probably on the insistence of his lawyer-father. Within two years, he completed his studies in both civil and canon law and passed the examination for the licentiate in law. This was to be the last of his formal education. He had no interest in practicing law and with a small inheritance, set about doing his "own thing" which led him, in spite of his tenuous health, to join the Dutch army in the spring of 1618. During this time, the only thing of note was his close friendship with Isaac Beeck, a mathematician and physician. René completed his military career unscathed. After leaving the army, he traveled throughout Europe for ten years, presumably rounding out his education, as was then the custom. On 11 November 1619, he had three dreams, which changed the course of his life. During one of these dreams, he opened a book that read, *Quod vitae sectabor iter?* (What road of life shall I take)? He prayed to God and received an "illumination" that revealed to him the *mirabilis scientiae fundamentia* (the wonderful foundations of science). Descartes tried to prove our existence and that of God with these principles. This divine illumination prompted him to promise a pilgrimage to the sanctuary of the Holy Virgin at San Loreto, Italy—a promise he did not immediately keep.

In 1624, three young men were banished from France for planning an anti-Aristotelian demonstration. Such action was potentially a capital offense. This may have led to Descartes' long self-imposed exile in Holland. His anti-Aristotelian sentiments were beginning to emerge and these ideas were tantamount to heresy. In the Low Countries, he lived a retiring but highly intellectual life, corresponding regularly with like-minded peers. He immersed himself in scientific and philosophical pursuits and, of course, writing. His first treatise was the *Discourse on Method*, published anonymously in 1637. He had an illegitimate son during this period, who died at age five of scarlet fever—a tragedy that affected him deeply. He carried on an extended correspondence with Princess Elizabeth, the daughter of the Winter King of Bohemia, that lasted for nearly seven years, until a month before his death in 1650. In 1649 he accepted an invitation from Christina of Sweden, to join her court. The climate may have been unsuited to Descartes who died the next year.

Descartes' Medicine

In Part VI of the *Discourse*, he condemns the current state of medical knowledge:

> I believe that it is in medicine [that truth] must be sought for. It is true that the science of medicine, as it now exists, contains few things whose utility is very remarkable: but without any wish to depreciate it, I am confident that there is no one, even among those whose profession it is, who does not admit that all present knowledge in medicine is almost nothing in comparison to what remains to be discovered; and that we could free ourselves from an infinity of maladies of body as well as of mind, and perhaps also even from the debility of age, if we had sufficiently ample knowledge of their causes, and of all the remedies provided for us by nature.[65]

In the same section, Descartes, however, finds hope in the method of reasoning that he has devised for finding truth, truth that is practical and useful for all humans. Using his method he:

> Perceived it to be possible to arrive at knowledge highly useful in life…to discover a practical [knowledge of] the force and action of fire, water, air the stars, the heavens, and all the other bodies that surround us, [and thus] we might also apply them in the same way to all the uses to which they are adapted, and thus render ourselves the lords and possessors of nature.[66]

By his method, he meant a rational, demonstrative process that approaches the certitude of mathematics. Beginning with his famous *Cogito ergo sum* (I think therefore I am), he believed it was possible to devise a system of thought that was rigidly logical and capable of yielding indisputable truth. He contrasted this to the speculative knowledge Aristotle believed in, which for Descartes was fundamentally flawed since it was not based on the laws of mathematics and physics:

> But as soon as I had acquired some general notions respecting physics, and beginning to make trial of them in various particular difficulties, had observed how far they can carry us, and how much they differ from the principles that have been employed up to the present time.[67]

He indicates that his method involves not only rational but practical aspects, that is, empirically acquired data. It is evident from the foregoing that Descartes is not opposed to principles that include natural astrology. He seems to accept at least three of the four elements of the Ancients (fire, air and earth) as well as the forces that the stars and other heavenly bodies bring to bear on Earth and its inhabitants.

Descartes believed that God was not a deceiver, therefore, whatever seemed to be "clear and distinct" to our reason must be true.

> Since God has given each of us a light for the distinguishing of the true from the false, I could not believe that I ought to remain content for a single moment with the opinion of others.[68]

It was this principle of clear and distinct reasoning that guided him in his approach to truth. It allowed him, he believed, to prove not only personal existence but the existence of God and soul as well.

Descartes speaks of the many blessings God has given humankind, the most important is:

> Preservation of health, which is without doubt, of all the blessings of this life, the first and fundamental one; for the mind is so intimately dependent upon the condition and relation of the organs of the body, that if any means can ever be found to render men wiser and more ingenious than hitherto, I believe that it is in medicine they must be sought for. [69]

True knowledge was acquired in this way. It followed that it is in the knowledge of nature, gained in this manner (and this included medical knowledge) that the well-being of humans is to be found. This knowledge was attained by studying nature and utilizing the clear and distinct reasoning with which God supplies us humans.

Descartes, in fact, ends his *Discourse* with the following:

> I have resolved to devote what time I may still have to live to no other occupation than that of endeavoring to acquire some knowledge of Nature, which shall be of such a kind as to enable us there from to deduce rules in medicine of greater certainty than those at present in use.[70]

He appears to be totally dedicated to applying his method to the science of medicine since in so doing, he offers the greatest benefit to humankind. And though he devotes his considerable intellect to a variety of pursuits including philosophy, mathematics and the natural sciences, there is no doubt that medicine was a major interest of his even though he never became a formally trained physician.

Descartes sought the company of and became friends with a number of physicians. As noted above, his grandfather and great grandfather were physicians. These physician-friends were apparently interested in Descartes' new method of reasoning, especially as it could be applied to making medicine a more exact discipline—one that offered certainty and security to both patient and doctor.

In his conversations with these medical men he learned of William Harvey's treatise on circulation, *De motu cordis,* and its significance for both medicine and science as a whole.[71] These relationships did not always flow smoothly due possibly to Descartes' fundamental personality or his lack of formal medical training. His first Dutch friend following his return to the Low Countries was a physician by the name of Isaac Beeckman, who was more a mathematician and scientist than doctor (he never practiced medicine). Others of his physician-friends, such as Vopiscus Plemp, were practicing doctors. Plemp was a Galenist and did not initially accept Harvey's ideas regarding circulation. Plemp records that he often found Descartes engaged in animal dissections, suggesting that the latter may have been repeating the errors that Galen had made centuries before. Though Descartes and his medical friends differed on a number of issues, both medical and philosophical, their association provided a milieu that fostered a variety of intellectual pursuits that benefited Descartes as well as his friends. Undoubtedly, his concerns with medicine were promoted by these intellectual contacts.

Descartes, as mentioned, was not a trained physician. This did not prevent him from acting as such. It is recorded that in consultation with one of his doctor- friends, Descartes examined the daughter of a friend who had curvature of the bones and required the services of a surgeon.[72] The outcome of his ministrations is not certain but it appears that his physician-friends respected Descartes' medical views.

Descartes' medical knowledge came from extensive reading of medical writings, and at one point he considered composing a short survey of medicine—a task never completed. When discussing medical topics, it was usual for him to carefully avoid mentioning the authors from whom he derived his information seeking more than his share of prestige for these ideas. He was, however, once forced to admit that he did not know how to cure even a fever.[73] In this failing, he was not alone. For much had been written about fevers dating to Hippocrates, but little, if anything, was available to the healer that could actually treat, no less cure, a fever.[74] Descartes studied chemistry and botany but in a very limited way and there is little evidence that he achieved any level of competence in either field.[75] Anatomy and embryology were another matter, for it appears that he dissected animals over an eleven-year period and later boasted that no physician knew anatomy better than he. It was claimed that he spent time watching butchers slaughter cattle, though he was hesitant to admit this. He apparently took parts of cattle from the butcher to study at home. He also attended lectures and public dissections of human cadavers at Leiden. He was especially interested in the pineal gland which he viewed as the seat of the soul. This "gland," he believed, was the location of the immortal soul and the connecting area in the brain between the body and soul. As such, it was anatomically central to his dualistic theory of human beings.

Aristotle, Thomas Aquinas, and Descartes

As we have seen, Descartes was trained by the Jesuits in Scholastic philosophy. As also noted earlier, Aristotle believed in the four elements of Empedocles and their associated qualities (hot, cold, wet, and dry). He also posited entelechy or *formis substantialis*. This substantial form "actualizes" prime matter to make a being what it is, which includes its purpose or teleology. The entelechy is also known as the soul. Aristotle and Thomas Aquinas believed there were three souls: vegetative, sensitive and rational. Plants had only the first, animals the first two and humans all three. In his view, the animal soul developed in the male on the fortieth day of fetal life and in the female on the eightieth day. Women were viewed as inferior to men and had a lesser kind of soul, according to Aristotle. The entire soul was not immortal in Aristotle's view, only the "active intellect." The soul, in a sense, has multiple parts. That the whole soul was not immortal was at odds with Catholic theology. Also, a spiritual entity should not have parts. Aristotle placed the human soul in the heart, along with innate heat. Neither sensation nor the soul was to be found in the brain. Aristotle wrote of these ideas in *De anima*.[76]

Thomas Aquinas (1225-1274) christianized Aristotle as Augustine of Hippo had done for Plato. Thomas differed from Aristotle on two major points: the world was not eternal and the soul was immortal. By these two alterations, Aristotle became theologically digestible by Church theologians and Aristotle largely replaced Plato as the philosopher of Catholicism.

Dualism

As noted, Descartes disavowed the Scholastics' approach to acquisition of knowledge—it was too speculative, non-empirical, and impractical.

The Scholastics spent all their time and energies speculating on how many angels could dance on the head of pin rather than what could help humans live better. In this sense, Descartes was a true humanist. Nonetheless, he viewed himself as a good Catholic. As with Galileo, he wanted orthodoxy but not empty truths contradicted by scientific evidence. He did not believe in orthodoxy at any cost. Scripture was not the only warrant for "truth."

A major problem for Descartes was the mind-body dualism of Aristotle, Thomas and the Catholic theology that flowed from them. Dualism, as opposed to monism, sees humans as consisting of soul and body—the one spiritual, the other physical. Monists see the mind-body dichotomy as nonexistent. Each was an aspect of one natural, physical principle. If one were a materialist, all could be explained on a purely physical basis. The workings of the brain explained what the dualists call the soul or mind. Others explain the soul as an epiphenomenon of the workings of the body and especially the brain. Matrialists claim that the soul or mind is an accidental by-product of brain activity. There are other theories offered to explain the mind-body dilemma but they can be reduced to one of the foregoing views.[77] Because of his religious views and his belief that God provides clear and distinct ideas based on reason and observation—God was not a deceiver— Descartes was convinced that there were these two principles within human nature. How a spiritual entity could affect a physical one was the issue for Descartes, the dualist. Since these two worlds were metaphysically distinct, they lay on either side of an unbridgeable abyss. Descartes attempted to span this chiasm by analogy. He compares the effect of Earth's gravity[78] on a stone to the effect a spiritual force can have on a body. Each was invisible and mysterious. Descartes saw a similarity between the two concepts. This, of course, explained nothing scientifically but allowed him a way to link the two principles.

Descartes' Neurophysiology and Psychology

The question arose in Descartes' mind as to where the soul was located in the body. Strictly speaking, a spiritual thing, since it is immaterial, existed in no space—space implies materiality—and all spirits are immaterial. This is inherent in the divide that separates the two realms of body and soul. Ignoring this difficulty, he plows forward in his quest to unite body and mind. The pineal gland is:

> Where the seat of imagination and common sense [and sensation] is, which should be taken to be ideas, that is to say, to be the forms of images that the rational soul will consider directly when, being united to this machine (the body), it will imagine or it will sense any objects.[79]

The functions of the *sensorius commune* included imagination, ideas, thinking, and perception via the five senses. Memory was not localized and involved many parts of the brain and even muscles. However, there was an "intellectual memory" that was separate from the more functional memory and this was found in the soul localized to the pineal gland. Descartes' scheme was an adaptation of Galen's neurophysiology, whereby the blood supplying the brain goes first to the pineal gland, then the ventricles of the brain, thereafter, to the spinal cord through the nerves (believed to be hollow) to the muscles and other tissues. The concept of circulation was just beginning to be propagated. Previous to this, blood was thought to move "to and fro" in the arteries and veins. Whether Descartes was thinking in terms of true circulation or swishing of blood, it somehow delivered what Descartes called "animal spirits" to the entire body. These spirits nourished and vitalized the body. He describes the animal spirit:

> As a certain very subtle wind, or rather a very lively and very pure flame.[80]

Whether the animal spirit is the vital heat or *pneuma* is not clear. But all the body must have access to it in order to carry on its vital functions. Descartes apparently believed all the blood from the heart goes to the pineal gland and thence to the brain and rest of the body. The soul then has a "view" of all the blood before it passes to the periphery. The soul must be seen as forming images and judgments but also impacting the workings of the body and, in turn being impacted by the body. This has to be a two-way street, in order to completely explain the body-mind interaction that appears to occur in health and disease.

Muscular and Digestive Physiology

Descartes develops a complex physiology to explain voluntary muscular movement. Princess Elizabeth of Bohemia actually stimulated Descartes' interest in this problem.[81] His answer did not satisfy the Princess and for good reason—it was flawed. He claimed that the union of mind and body was a "primary notion." The soul is of such a character that it can be unified with the body. A tautology if there ever was one. It begs the question, giving no substantial explanation. It says nothing, answers nothing and smacks of the empty Scholasticism that so annoyed

Descartes. Even if we grant that the soul exists and has an innate power, the question still remains: how does an immaterial being connect with a material being so that this power can be utilized to cause change in a physical being?

The animal spirits were "fire without flames" that nourished and vivified all parts of the body. However, this fire could go awry at times and become localized causing erysipelas,[82] abscesses, fevers, or other inflammatory conditions. Disease in general was considered to result from mechanical failure of the machine (body); this is not well delineated by Descartes, however.

Digestion occurred by trituration and coction, both reminiscent of Galen's scheme. These were mediated by heating food in the gastrointestinal tract. It was commonly held in Antiquity that heat mediated the work of digestion. Digestive enzymes were, of course, unknown. However, Descartes did posit some humors that catalyzed this process. In this, he moved a step beyond Galen's system but still it was a speculative step not verified by experimentation. The heat, along with the motion of the intestines, "agitated" and broke up the food making it ready to be transported through pores in the intestinal wall to the blood, then to the heart where it is further heated, moving on to the brain as noted above.[83]

The animal spirits account for muscle contraction.[84] The nerves again serve as conduits to transport the animal spirits to the muscles. These spirits have already passed through the pineal gland where the "imagination" of the soul has directed the spirits to their proper terminus, in this case the muscles. Where the nerves enter the muscles there are small valves that open allowing the spirits to flow in with great force causing the muscles to swell, that is, contract. This process is not active. The muscles are made to swell and do not do so of their own accord. Relaxation of the muscles occurs when another set of valves opens, allowing the spirits to escape and the muscle to shrink and soften. How the valves are opened or closed is not specified. All of Descartes' Universe is a mechanistic system but many aspects of his system go unexplained.

Descartes believed in Fire as the vital principle in all bodily functions. He also accepted Air and Earth as two other "elements."[85] Water was not included among his "elements." The "particles" consisted of one, two or three elements. These particles were further classified by size, shape, and motion (or lack thereof). The Sun and stars were composed of only Fire. The "heavens" outside the Sun and stars consists of mostly Air with Fire filling the "interstices" between.

The Earth, planets and comets were made up of three-element particles. These three types of matter were "pure," that is, the elements within them were of the same size, shape, and motion. Material things of the Earth, however, including living and non-living things, are composed of "mixed" particles. The constituent elements including Fire, Air and Earth—vary in size, shape, and motion. This structure was necessary because Descartes' Universe was totally mechanistic. There was no void as the Atomists thought. Every particle was in contact with its neighboring particles. The world functioned as a vast series of pushes and pulls. This system did not recognize chemistry or biology, only physics. The humoral theory, so long the bedrock of medicine, was essentially ignored by René Descartes. Even though he admits to three elements, their role in health and disease is strictly physical. Fire plays a role in disease but not the other three elements of Empedocles. Of the four qualities, only heat was of concern. Except for blood, the humors were ignored and this humor was only of use in its ability to carry heat and animal spirits. In essence, Descartes bade Hippocrates, Aristotle, and Galen a silent farewell.

Descartes' impact on medicine and his influence on the development of modern medicine were not decisive. Nonetheless, his ideas and how he applied them to medicine made a difference to those that followed him. He recognized that the Ancients had developed a largely speculative system. Their mental machinations were interesting intellectual endeavors and certainly helped philosophers and other thinkers including medical men and women, to gradually cast a rational, systematic, if flawed light on the darkness in which the mysteries of nature were shrouded. His anti-Aristotelianism was one of the earliest blows aimed at this beloved ancient philosophical system. The very fact that he found it necessary to immigrate to Holland to avoid ecclesiastical and secular sanctions, speaks to the sacrosanct nature of Scholastic thought at the time. His ideas were significant milestones on the road to modern medicine.

In addition, his mechanistic view of the world was important in toppling the highly rationalized humoral system of Galen. Again, even though this scheme contained certain biological and chemical features that may have been applied to the "new" medicine, the fact is that the humoral system did not trend this way. A revolution in chemistry and the biological sciences was necessary to eventually turn the corner onto modern medicine. Descartes' physical, mechanical world ultimately failed to explain the medical world but at least it helped shift the focus from Galen, allowing new paradigms to emerge. Descartes' empiricism was sorely lacking in true science. His anatomy was little more than Galen-ism warmed over (if one can use this mixed metaphor). His dissections only led to more speculative, unsubstantiated theories. It was hardly even anecdotal in nature. He used his animal anatomy mainly to reinforce his preconceived ideas of medicine. Steelehall suggests that Descartes "applied his broad assumptions with a kind of deductive blindness, and a disregard for verification."[86] In spite of these criticisms, Descartes was not only a great intellect but also a man of moral strength who stood up to the forces that wished to maintain the status quo.

Isaac Newton

Isaac Newton (1642-1727 C.E.) further diminished Aristotle's cred-ibility when he developed his laws of motion.[87] Aristotle had maintained that objects thrust into the air persisted in motion by some "helping hand" or "impetus" that continually pushed the object along until it ultimately fell to Earth, Aristotle asserted that all material bodies "naturally"[88] migrated toward the Earth.[89] The heavenly bodies all moved unendingly in circles—such motion was the most perfect form of motion—earthly bodies followed a "rectilinear" motion, which was straight and always tended toward the ground. Fire and air "naturally" moved upward in a rectilinear fashion but water and earth naturally sought the lower reaches of the globe. Newton, however, proclaimed that all bodies, earthly or ce-lestial, moved in a straight line unless acted upon by some outside force. Such bodies had no "natural" direction in which they moved. Material things moved toward Earth only because of the gravitational pull of Earth. Where there was no gravity, they would simply go on their merry way until affected by some outside force. This force could be gravity, friction or impact with another body. With these laws, Newton further weakened Aristotle's authority, which had been the basis for all natural sciences, including medicine, for so many centuries. In addition to these insults to Aristotle, (and Galen) there were to be added experimental medical findings that directly impugned the veracity of these long-honored men. The findings of Copernicus, Brahe, Galileo, Newton, and other early scientists, though not medical in nature, nonetheless, raised serious questions about the authority of the Ancients. Medical researchers were to add their own evidence that was to undercut the now wobbly struts supporting medieval medicine.

Notes

1.   Crowe, M. J. 1990, *Theories of the World from Antiquity to the Copernican Revolution* (New York: Dover).
2.   Heath, T. L. 1991. *Greek Astronomy*, p. 2.
3.   Ibid., p. 4.
4.   Ibid., pp. 3-5.
5.   Heraclitus, 2003, *Fragments*, trans. B. Haxton (New York: Penguin), p. xii.
6.   Lambridis, H. 1976. *Empedocles*, p. 31.
7.   Guthrie, K. S. 1988. *Pythagorean Source Book*, pp. 61-63.
8.   Heath, T. L. 1991. *Greek Astronomy*, p. 61.
9.   Wright, M. R. 1995, *Empedocles: The Extant Fragments* (Indianapolis, IN: Hackett), pp. 9-14.
10. Clegg, B. 2003, *The First Scientist: A Life of Roger Bacon* (New York: Carroll & Graf).
11. Witzel, T. 2003, *Catholic Encyclopedia* XIII (New York: Online Edition).
12. Latin translations of Aristotle's writings had just begun to penetrate Europe in the twelfth century and the "Christianizing" of "The Philosopher" was barely beginning.
13. Clegg, B. 2003. The First *Scientist: A Life of Roger Bacon* (New York: Carroll & Graff), p. 113.
14. Thatcher, O. J. 1901, *The Library of Original Sources* (Milwaukee, WI: University Research Extension). Internet Medieval Source Book.
15. Bacon, R. 1998, *Opus majus*, trans. R. Belle (New York: Kesinger), p. 583.
16. Ibid., p. 584.
17. Ibid.
18. A stone once believed to be impenetrable due to its hardness.
19. Ibid., p. 385.
20. Ibid., p. 582. Bacon suggests that Julius Caesar used a series of mirrors to spy on the Britons from Gaul.
21. McEvoy, J. 2000, *Robert Grosseteste* (New York: Oxford University Press), p. 88.
22. Ibid., pp. 410-581.
23. Ibid., p. 582.
24. Wilson, C. 1980, *The Starseekers* (Garden City, NY: Doubleday & Co.), p. 123.
25. Anton van Leeuwenhoek has been given credit for inventing the microscope though some have attributed this feat to Galileo.
26. Clegg. 2003. The First Scientist, pp. 156-157.
27. Bramly, S. 1994, *Leonardo: The Artist and the Man*, trans. S. Reynolds (London: Penguin), p. xi.
28. Ibid., p. 5.
29. Nicholl, C. 2004, *Leonardo da Vinci: Flights of the Mind* (London: Viking Penguin), p. 155.
30. Leonardo may have been the first to suggest that seashells found on mountain tops arrived there while under the ocean, later to be elevated by geological forces yet to be discovered, that is, tectonic uplifting.
31. Ibid., p. 240.
32. Da Vinci, L. 1983, *Leonardo on the Human Body*, trans. & text, O'Malley, C.D. and Saunders, J.B. de C.M. (New York: Dover), p. 13.
33. Ibid. These authors suggest that the bull, *De sepulturus*, issued by Pope Boniface VIII in 1300, proscribing boiling of human bones (in order to preserve them for transportation) did not disallow human dissection.

34. Ibid.
35. Bramly, S. 1994. *Leonardo*, pp. 12-13. There is evidence that most of the thirty autopsies were observed and only five or six actually performed by da Vinci.
36. Nicholl, C. 2004. *Leonardo da Vinci*, p. 242.
37. Da Vinci, L. 2005, *Leonardo's Notebooks*, ed. H. Anna Suh (New York: Black Dog & Leventhal), p. 149.
38. Harvey was to show that blood circulated at a much higher rate making continuous blood production at this higher rate unlikely. One could not consume enough food to keep up with the demand for newly produced blood.
39. Da Vinci, L. 1983. *Leonardo on the Human Body*, pp. 216-220.
40. Ibid., p. 21.
41. Blood is not produced in the liver but in the bone marrow. It circulates through the liver to the hepatic vein to the inferior vena cava to the right atrium, right ventricle and to the lungs via the pulmonary artery, back to the heart via the pulmonary vein into the left atrium, left ventricle then out the aorta to the rest of the body. The two ventricles contract simultaneously, rather than alternately, as Leonardo believed.
42. Da Vinci, L. 2005. *Leonardo's Notebooks*, p. 150.
43. Ibid., p. 167.
44. Tufa: The calcareous and siliceous rock deposits of springs, lakes, or ground water.
45. Ibid., p. 168.
46. Nicholl, C. 2004. *Leonardo da Vinci*, p. 245.
47. Da Vinci, L. 2005. *Leonardo's Notebooks*, p. 4.
48. Nicholl, C. 2004, p. 245.
49. A canon was an unordained clergyman who attended to many of the day-to-day functions of the cathedral and lived a celibate, semi-monastic life with the other canons stationed at the church he served.
50. Rosen, E. 1984, *Copernicus and the Scientific Revolution* (Malabar, FL: Robert E. Krieger).
51. Copernicus, N. 1995, *On the Revolutions of Heavenly Spheres* (Amherst, NY: Prometheus Books).
52. Ibid., p. 3.
53. Ptolemy 1998, *Almagest*, trans. G. J. Toomer (Princeton, NJ: Princeton University Press).
54. Copernicus, N. 1995. *On the Revolutions*, p. 9.
55. Aristarchus (c. 217-c. 145 B.C.E.) had proposed a heliocentric system but gained few adherents.
56. Ibid., p. 11.
57. Christianson, J. R. 2000, *On Tycho's Island: Tycho Brahe and his Assistants, 1590-1601* (New York: Cambridge University Press) p. 17.
58. Ibid., pp. 17-18. The supernova appeared in the constellation Cassiopeia.
59. Garber, J. J. 2002, "Cepheid Variables: A Philosophical and Scientific Odyssey," University of Western Sydney, History of Astronomy Paper.
60. Ibid.
61. Astrometry is the measurement of the positions of stars.
62. The third law states that the time it takes a planet to revolve around the Sun squared is equal to its mean distance from the Sun cubed. $P^2=d^3$.
63. Galilei, G. 1957, "Starry Messenger," trans. S. Drake in *Discoveries and Opinions of Galileo* (Garden City, NY: Doubleday-Anchor). These moons are Io, a volcanically active satellite that spews out noxious gases; Europa, thought to harbor vast

stretches of surface ice with watery sludge beneath this surface. A satellite probe to Europa is planned in the near future. The outer two moons, Ganymede and Calypso, are the largest of the four Jovian moons.

64. It is very unusual for two "naked-eye" supernovae to be observed so close together in time.
65. Lindboom, G.A. 1979, *Descartes and Medicine* (Amsterdam: Rodopi), p. 2.
66. Descartes, R. 1958, *Descartes' Philosophical Writings, Discourse on Method*, trans. N. K. Smith (New York: The Modern Library, Random House), p. 131.
67. Ibid., p. 130.
68. Ibid.
69. Ibid., p. 115.
70. Ibid., p. 131.
71. Ibid., p. 143.
72. Lindboom, G. A. 1978, *Descartes and Medicine*.
73. Lindboom, G. A. 1978, pp. 29, 33.
74. Ibid., p. 36.
75. Hippocrates. 1978. *Hippocratic Writings*, pp. 80-82.
76. Op. cit. Lindboom, G. A. 1979, p. 36.
77. Aristotle. 1984, *De Anima*. pp. 641-692.
78. Kalat, J. W. 1992, *Biological Psychology*, 4th edition (Belmont, CA: Wadsworth), p. 11.
79. Gravity was not to be defined until later in the seventeenth century by Newton but it was evident from the time of Aristotle that something caused objects to fall to the ground. Aristotle assigned this to "natural inclinations" of sublunary bodies to move toward the center of the globe.
80. Descartes, R. 2003. *Treatise of Man*, trans. T. Steelehall (Amherst, NY: Prometheus Books), p. 86.
81. Ibid., p. 19.
82. Op. cit. Lindboom, G. A. 1979, p. 57.
83. An inflammatory condition of the skin usually caused by the *Streptococcus* bacterium.
84. Descartes, R. 2003. *Treatise of Man*, pp. 5-9.
85. Ibid., pp. 21-25.
86. Ibid., p. 2.
87. Ibid., p. xxvii.
88. Newton, I. 1934, *Principia*: Vol. I, *The Motion of Bodies* (Berkeley: University of California Press).
89. It was in the "nature" of earthy objects to move to Earth. It had nothing to do with gravity—this rectilinear motion was a metaphysical characteristic of sublunary objects according to Aristotle.
90. Aristotle 1984, *Physics, The Complete Works of Aristotle* (Princeton, NJ: Princeton University Press).

7

Medicine on the Mend

Paracelsus: the Father of Iatrochemistry

Theophrastus Philippus Aureolus Bombastus von Hohenheim (c. 1493-1542 C.E.), later known as Paracelsus, is considered by many to be the Father of iatrochemistry.[1] Iatrochemistry, from the Greek "doctor's chemistry," involves the use of chemicals in the treatment of disease, as opposed to herbal remedies employed in the practice of medicine for so many millennia. Paracelsus[2] considered himself the epitome of modern medical practitioners and with his arrogant manner managed to alienate most of the physicians of his day. The name, Paracelsus, meaning "surpassing Celsus," [3] was indicative of his perceived superiority as a physician. Paracelsus demeaned Hippocratic medicine as pure speculation and not worthy of the label "science." Today, Paracelsus' works are considered, at best, medically marginal. He wrote on hermetic astronomy and medicine[4] and was taught medicine primarily by his physician-father, attending medical school only briefly. Subsequently, he became a wandering healer.[5] His medicine was heavily influenced by mystical and magical elements. He was convinced that there were invisible powers intermediate between God and man, providing humans with God's divine healing power. Though a Catholic throughout his life, he was "Protestant" in his outlook, eschewing Church authority, as well as the authority of the Ancients, such as Aristotle and Galen. He proclaimed that empirically based medicine was essential; nonetheless, he persisted in revising speculative theories about science and specifically medicine.

> When I saw that nothing resulted from (doctors') practice but killing and suffering, I determined to abandon such a miserable art and seek truth elsewhere."[6]

It was in his willingness to break with the Galenic tradition of medicine that Paracelsus is most notable. His theory of medicine was, in fact, just as speculative as that of the practitioners who preceded him.

He did, however, promote iatrochemistry, which opened a new therapeutic path for medicine. Rather than the four humors as a basis for his medical theory, he separated all substances into "sulfur," "mercury" and "salt." These were not considered to be material elementst, rather "hidden powers" that gave earthly objects their material characteristics. Paracelsus saw Nature as sovereign and the physician's role was to understand and obey her rules. He put great stock in folk remedies as arising out of the knowledge of Nature and saw Nature as "illegible" to proud university professors but evident to pious adepts.

This knowledge of Nature draws upon the "doctrine of signatures" as a sign of the curative power of various remedies. For example, the orchid looks like a testicle (the name orchid comes from the Greek for testicle) and thus had an ability to heal venereal diseases. The plant, eyebright, had been made by Nature to resemble a blue eye, as an indication that it could be used to treat eye disorders. Paracelsus may have been influenced by radical Protestantism, in which the priesthood was inherent in all people so too, was medical knowledge. Truth was not found in musty folios but in the forests and fields and in the heart. He proudly proclaimed, "I tell you one hair on my neck knows more than all you authors (university professors), and my shoe-buckles contain more wisdom than both Galen and Avicenna."

In 1526, he was appointed town physician and professor of medicine at Basal. This required that he lecture to the medical faculty, which he did, but not in academic robes, as was the custom. Instead, he wore an alchemist's leather apron, delivering lectures in German, not Latin. From the outset, he proclaimed that he would not teach Hippocrates and Galen since experience alone is enough to disclose the secrets of disease. All of these insults did not endear him to the academics of Basel, though he was loved by the students, always eager for a battle with the establishment. He publicly burned Avicenna's *Canons of Medicine*, one of the most revered medical texts of the day. He subjected several of Hippocrates' writings to the same treatment.

Paracelsus' significance lies in his emphasis on chemical principles of medicine.[7] For him, sulfur was the fiery principle in matter, mercury, its "spiritousness" or volatility and salt, its solidity and consistency. He did not entirely reject the four qualities, elements and humors but saw his tripartite system as representing the "male" aspect of Nature as "active and spiritual," whereas the traditional Aristotelian-Galenic elements as "female and passive."

He associated diseases with the spirits of certain minerals and metals. Erysipelas[8] was induced by vitriol[9] and cancer by "colcothar" (ferrous peroxide). He employed metals and minerals, such as mercury, antimony, iron, arsenic, lead, copper, and sulfur, therapeutically, often in large doses.[10] He believed that living processes were based on two chemical principles. The first he called *archei,* which was an internal living property that controlled vital functions, such as digestion. The second principle was *semina* or seeds, derived from God, the great orchestrator of Nature. This principle was responsible for reproduction and generative processes such as growth and development. God employed a great Alchemist (one of Paracelsus' intermediaries between God and humans) to do His bidding in this scheme.[11] Disease, on the other hand, emanated from two sources: stellar toxins (this would include the stars, planets and comets as the sources of these toxins) in a classical astrological sense.[12] The second source was from earthly minerals, especially certain salts. Each disease had a specific external cause and these causes were manifold. He suggested that arsenic itself was responsible for 100 distinct diseases.[13] In the end, such causes were not so much material as spiritual or metaphysical, in the sense that they were speculative and not empirically derived. In spite of the criticism of the Galenic theory of medicine, his approach smacks of the Ancients and their often magical theories of disease.

Diagnostically, he rejected the inspection of urine (uroscopy) and the other classical methods of defining etiology, in favor of alchemical means using distillation and coagulation tests. He viewed dissection as worthless "dead anatomy," which tells us nothing about living, bodily functions. Determining abnormal quantities of sulfur, mercury or salt was of more diagnostic value than postulating imbalances of the four humors. How Paracelsus measured the levels of sulfur, mercury or salt is uncertain.[14]

Hippocrates viewed gouty arthritis as an imbalance of the humors—a "defluxion" into the foot. Gutta (gout) means flowing, Paracelsus, on the other hand, saw gout as a chemical problem classified as a "tartaric disease," that is, a disease of "incrustation."[15] Some mineral was being deposited in the foot causing the arthritis.[16] This mineral might come from various sources, including food and the local water supply. Other tartaric diseases were gallstones, kidney stones, and dental plaques, still referred to as tartar today. He viewed Switzerland, his homeland, as a very healthy country. Again, his ideas seem to echo the speculative biases of Hippocrates[17] and Aristotle.[18]

Although Porter sees Paracelsus as a "breath of fresh air" that was the "inspiration for the new medicine emerging during the early "scientific revolution," this would seem to be a stretch. His ideas were far from "scientific" in the modern, empirical sense and, though diverging from the long-held theories of the Ancients, they brought little new to medicine besides their emphasis on chemistry (one might even say alchemy). His sulfur, mercury and salt are little more than a restatement of the humoral theory. It is recognized today that chemistry plays a role in the causation and cure of certain diseases but not in the metaphysical sense that Paracelsus proposed.[19] Arsenic does cause a specific disease syndrome but not a 100 different diseases. The same can be said for mercury and lead. Paracelsus has certainly captured the imagination of present day scholars and provides fodder for practitioners of alternative medicine but it is difficult to place him in the role of a major reformer of medicine. Albertus Magnus in the thirteenth century and others before him may have advocated the use of various minerals in the treatment of disease,[20] but the use of "stones," minerals and earthy substances, such as calamine, date to Antiquity and are not the invention of Paracelsus.

In all fairness, it must be said that Paracelsus was not without significant influence during the transition from medieval to modern medicine.[21] He recognized that change came from outside the body and was not necessarily endogenous in origin—relating to the four humors. This was an important concept though not entirely novel. Both Hippocrates and Aristotle were aware of this, though in their system it was the humors that ultimately mediated health and disease. For Paracelsus, sulfur, mercury, and salt seem to have replaced the humors. The two systems are otherwise similar. His most significant notion may rest with the idea of universal change. The superlunary Universe was not fixed as the Ancients had claimed and this cosmological insight may have influenced Tycho Brahe's interpretation of the supernova of 1572 and the impact this had on undermining Aristotle's authority, which ultimately led to an entirely new scientific paradigm. How pivotal Paracelsus' ideas were in the overall transformation of medical theory is uncertain but bears inclusion in our present discussion of medical modernization.

Andreas Vesalius

Andreas Vesalius (1514-1564 C.E.) could be considered the first true innovator of medical thought in the early Enlightenment. He was born Andreas van Wesele in Brussels, where his father was pharmacist to the Holy Roman Emperor, Charles V. Preferring the Latinized form of his family name, he is known as Vesalius.[22] After studying Latin and Greek as a youth, Vesalius enrolled in the Faculty of Medicine at the University of Paris, mentored by the conservative humanist, Sylvius, who was an advocate of Galenic medicine and anatomy. Sylvius later said Vesalius was a "madman," apparently because of his intense devotion to anatomical dissection. Legend has it he once robbed a wayside gibbet[23] in order to obtain anatomic material. In 1536, war forced him to flee Paris and return to Louvain University, in present day Belgium, where he introduced his refined dissecting techniques that he had learned from Guinther von Andernach. The next year, moving to Padua, one of the most prestigious

Figure 7.1
Vesalius' Humanistic Depiction of a Human Skeleton

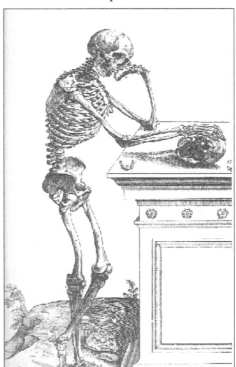

medical schools of the period, he developed a reputation as a talented anatomist. Dissection had previously been demonstrated by surgeons (who were considered inferior to physicians) consequently, the subject had not been a required course for medical students.

The rediscovery of Galen's *On Anatomical Procedures* and his *On the Use of Parts*, as well as the growing humanist movement, stirred an interest in anatomical studies among fledgling physicians. Academics were becoming more interested in humankind and less so in speculative and spiritual pursuits. A focus on the human body was a natural consequence of humanism.[24]

Vesalius was, at heart, a Galenist, following Galen's dictum to "see for himself" when studying human anatomy. In spite of this devotion to Galen, Vesalius was his most open critic. Few anatomists, up to that time, were willing to find fault with the Master's view of the human body. Galen had dissected animals only, and, as noted above, this resulted in a number of anatomical errors, including the depiction of a five-lobed liver and a heart like that of an ape. In fact, in Vesalius' earliest illustrations he included these errors, later correcting them.

Vesalius' major work was, *De humani corporis fabrica* (On the fabric of the human body), published first in 1543. It has been pointed out by Charles Singer, writing on the occasion of the 400th anniversary of the publication of Vesalius' *Fabrica* that this term is not to be understood as a lifeless "fabric" or structure, but, rather, as an active, ongoing artistic endeavor—as something actively working or functioning—in a physiological rather than a unchanging anatomical icon.[25] Galen's, *On the Use of Parts*, is a textbook of physiology, not anatomy, and Vesalius wanted to emphasize the body as a dynamic, active entity rather than the "dead anatomy" denounced by Paracelsus. The *Fabrica* is also remarkable for its sophisticated art. The majority of illustrations were not done by Vesalius rather by a student of the famous Italian Renaissance artist, Titian, a certain Jan Stephan van Calcar (1499-c. 1546).[26] With the emergence of humanistic ideas of action and human vitality, along with the techniques of perspective, using the woodblock engravings that were created for the *Fabrica,* Vesalius was able to introduce a new liveliness and reality to the world of anatomy (see figures 7.1).

As we have seen, Galen dissected animals including pigs and apes, extrapolating these finding to humans, thus introducing errors that were to persist for 1,500 years. Vesalius, however, took pains to find human cadavers to autopsy. The word autopsy, in fact, means "to see for oneself." He was not limited by his respect for Galen and openly exposed the Master's mistakes. As an example, Vesalius realized that there was no *rete mirabile*[27] in the human brain as there was in some lower animals. He also recognized that the human liver was normally bi-lobed, not composed of five lobes as in the ape. Also, the human heart differed from that of the lower primates.[28] These findings made it clear that Galen had only dissected animals and his findings contained many errors. Vesalius then began to challenge Galen on a number of issues. The human mandible was found to consist of a single bone, not two, as in apes. In 1539, he acquired a supply of cadavers from executed convicts. It was his studies on these specimens that led to the *Fabrica*. After completing the woodcuts created in the studio of Titian, he personally carried them over the Alps from Venice to Basel in 1542, where the printer, Johannes Oporinus, published the *Fabrica* the next year. Vesalius provided a commentary for each woodcut and these included exact descriptions of the skeleton, muscles, nervous system, arteries, veins, and viscera.

Vesalius' work was not so remarkable for the number of Galen's errors that he exposed, rather for providing a systematic critique of the Master, pointing out that Galen had not used human cadavers, even though he wanted the reader to think so. In the process, Vesalius produced the first comprehensive anatomical study of the human body. Galen had been an egotistical showman, placing himself above all other physicians of his time.[29] He was given to holding public displays of his medical knowledge in order to impress both aristocrat and commoner, as well as, other physicians. These antics, as noted above, gained him a position as physician to the Emperor, Marcus Aurelius.[30] Along with his extensive writings this established him as the foremost physician since Hippocrates and made him the single most credible authority up to the Enlightenment. This hold on the medieval mind is best expressed by Ioannes Argenterius (1513-1573):

> The philosophers want it that Aristotle, uniquely, never erred. The physicians fight for Galen, and everyone most zealously battles for his author, without any shame.[31]

It was not Vesalius alone who undermined the long-held authority of Galen. Human dissection had been out of vogue since the anatomical work carried out in Alexandria in the third century b.c.e.[32] Herophilus and Erasistratus, separately, performed dissections of the human body, the former of the viscera and eye, the latter, the brain. Subsequently, study of the human cadaver declined for religious reasons and it was not until the late Middle Ages that physicians began to carry out autopsies in order to determine the cause of death in their patients. This trend allowed Vesalius to begin his dissections that led eventually to the downfall of, not only the authority of Galen, but Aristotle, along with their entire theory of medicine. This was not a sudden event; it took time and research in other disciplines to complete the transformation. One physician central to the evolution of modern medicine was William Harvey.

William Harvey

William Harvey (1578-1657 c.e.) was an April Fool's baby who proved to be anything but a fool and is one of the most influential physician-physiologist of all time.[33] His discovery of the true nature of circulation in the human body, more than any other medical finding, proved to be the most devastating denial of medieval medical theory. He was born the first of nine children of Thomas Harvey and his second wife, Joan Hawke Harvey. His father was elected mayor of Folkstone near Dover in 1587, just before the Spanish Armada was to encounter the English navy in 1588—a major turning point in the military history of England. Upon entering Canterbury Grammar School, he was described as a "spirited" youth possessed of a charitable disposition and what was to be a lifelong, quiet loyalty to the Anglican faith. His mother seems to have been responsible for these traits. From his father he inherited a vigor and capacity for hard work. He learned Latin and Greek and, in due course, entered Caius College, Cambridge, There he earned the Matthew Parker medical scholarship and spent his next six years in pursuit of a medical degree. He left Cambridge in 1599, believing, as the Ancients had, that study abroad was crucial to a proper career. He went to Padua to study anatomy under Fabricius, one of the leading anatomists of the time. It was during this period that he showed an ability to do experimental research based on imaginative hypotheses and observational verification. The anatomy taught at Padua followed the principles that Vesalius had established in the sixteenth century. In 1602, Harvey received his Doctor of Medicine degree. It was in this year that Fabricius published a book on valves in the veins. (*De venarum ostiolis*). Harvey had done some research on vein valves while studying under Fabricius and this may have been where his interest in circulation began. Harvey returned to England convinced that:

> Careful observation is needed in every discipline, and sensation itself is often to be consulted. One's own experience is to be relied upon not that of someone else.[34]

This admonition was obviously one of the principles of the Enlightenment that was beginning to bring down the medicine of the previous ages. He also cautioned against accepting the authority of prior practitioners. He acknowledged Aristotle's belief that "all men naturally wish to know" but in order to know the natural world, it is necessary to "see for oneself" the truth of any premise—past or present. He decried the tendency of scientists, "inquiring into not what things are but rather what others have said about things." [35]

Whereas Vesalius subverted Galen's anatomy, it remained for Harvey to do the same to Galen's physiology. In the 1600s, the accepted explanation for the origin of blood and its function in the human body was based on the concept of the four humors.[36] In traditional Aristotelian-Galenic physiology, there were two types of blood: venous and arterial, each with its own pathways and role in the three major centers of the body. These centers were the liver, responsible for nutrition and growth; the heart, which provides the body's vitality and warmth; and the brain, responsible for sensation and reason. Nutrition and growth resulted from the venous blood that originated in the liver. Food was transported from the gut to the liver, where new blood was manufactured, on a continual basis. Vitality came from the arterial blood, which was made in the heart. Arterial blood contained our old friend, *pneuma*,[37] which was "spirituous air," and this accounted for the vitality of the body. Both the venous and arterial blood, after providing their nutritional and vital functions, were then "used up" and did not return to the heart or liver. In this system, the blood was not considered to circulate throughout the body—it simply made its way to where needed and then was dissipated. The heart was not considered by Galen to be a pump. It simply sucked blood in during diastole—systole performed no significant function. The arterial movement of blood was explained by an innate "pulsative faculty" located in the arteries themselves. At best, the blood was thought of as swishing back and forth in the arteries.

A major feature of Galen's physiology lay in its explanation of the source of *pneuma*. Venous blood was mixed with *pneuma* in the left ventricle. This meant that venous blood had to somehow pass from the right to the left ventricle, in order to receive the *pneuma* provided by the heart. Galen posited "pores" in the interventricular septum through which the blood passed. The lungs were believed to cool the body. No thought of a pulmonary vascular circulation was entertained by the Ancients. Blood was "hot" in the Aristotelian-Galenic system and, since too much heat in the body would cause disease, there needed to be some form of "air conditioning" in the body to prevent overheating, and this was provided by the lungs. The air breathed into the lungs was conveyed to the left side of the heart for this purpose. The air was thought to reach the left ventricle via the pulmonary veins and, in turn, this air removed "sooty vapors" from the body during exhalation. The pulmonary veins provided a two-way street for these functions—air in, "sooty vapors" out. The failure to observe the living body, along with their penchant for specula-tion, accounts, in part at least, for the persistent belief in this system of respiration. In addition, the four humors and qualities seemed to fit well with this hypothesis. If the body produced too much blood and became hot, the lungs could bring in more air to cool the blood, thus accounting for rapid breathing when a person is over heated. If the body was too cool, it was assumed that it would compensate by producing more blood. Because blood was made from ingested food, if the wrong foods were consumed, disease could result. Proper diet would then restore the bal-ance of humors and qualities. Hippocrates had sanctioned eating more in winter in order to produce more blood and, therefore, more warmth for the body.[38] It all made perfect sense and given that authority was so esteemed in the Middle Ages, such concepts were to die hard. For cen-turies, the "pores" in the heart's interventricular septum, proposed by Galen, were to be sought in vain. In the second edition of the *Fabrica*, Vesalius questions the existence of these "pores."

Realdo Colombo (c.1515-1559) subsequently defined the anatomy and physiology of the pulmonary vascular tree and the role of left ventricular contractions (systole) in cardiac function.[39] He noted that the left ventricle discharged blood into the arteries and, that they then felt full—a critical finding for Harvey's later work. Andrea Casalpino (1519-1603) confirmed the function of the pulmonary vessels in "circulating" blood to the heart and lungs, described the function of the heart valves and began to use the term "circulation." In 1603, as noted earlier, Fabricius, Harvey's mentor, described the valves of the veins. All these observations came to final fruition in 1628, when Harvey published the *Excercitatio anatomica de motu cordis et sanguinis in animalibus* (An Anatomical Essay Concern-ing the Movement of the Heart and Blood in Animals). It is curious that Harvey used "neo-Aristotelian" methods to undermine the teachings of Aristotle. The latter had advocated the use of observation in studying nature but, in fact, had slipped into the traditional speculative mode of the ancient Greeks. Galen had fallen into the same error, observing dogs, apes, and pigs rather than humans.

The *De motu cordis* is divided into two parts. Harvey first points out several errors in Galen's anatomy. For instance, he notes that it would be hard to keep the incoming air and blood, which Galen said passed through the pulmonary vein, separate from the "sooty vapors" that passed out by the same route. Harvey put his criticism this way:

> [the pulmonary vein] will receive at one and the same time for two opposing purposes both blood and air, both warmth and cooling, which is improbable. [40]

Thus he denied for the first time that vessels carried blood at one moment and air at another. He observed no air in the pulmonary vein (or pulmonary artery) but only blood, in contrast to what the Ancients had maintained.[41] The second part of *De motu cordis* deals with the discovery of circulation. The "wisdom" of the centuries held that the only motion of blood was a "to and fro" movement of the blood but no true circulation, that is, no circuit of blood from the heart to the periphery and back again to the heart. The blood was believed to be used up and more had to be continually produced by the liver. In chapter six of *De motu cordis*, Harvey presents observations verifying the existence of a circulatory system in humans.[42] He first notes, in speaking of the flow of blood from arteries to veins to heart that:

> Were they [the Galenists] as experienced in the dissection of [living] animals as they are practiced in the anatomy of the dead human subject, this matter which keeps all involved in uncertainty would, in my view, be simply and readily clarified.[43]

He describes the pulmonary and peripheral circulation of a number of lower animals both cold and warm blooded, with, and without lungs (such as fishes). All of these *in vivo* observations demonstrated circulation of the blood. He showed this to be true as well in fetuses and embryos[44] He accurately describes the anatomy of the hepatic vein and its relationship to the vena cava, which had been misrepresented by Galen.[45]

Harvey defines the pulmonary circulation as follows:

> I maintain that in the more perfect and warmer animals…(as in man), the blood definitely penetrates the right ventricle of the heart through the artery-like [pulmonary] vein into the lungs, thence through the vein-like [pulmonary] artery into the left auricle, thence again into the left ventricle of the heart. I maintain, firstly, that this can happen, secondly, that it has so happened.[46]

Harvey not only lays out the physiology of the pulmonary vasculature, but also notes that the pulmonary artery (arteries carry blood away from the heart and veins toward the heart) actually is, anatomically, a vein and the pulmonary vein, an artery. Oxygenated blood generally leaves the heart and un-oxygenated blood enters the heart. This is the one situation in the body where the reverse is true. And, as mentioned, he finds no visible air in the pulmonary vessels. He reviews these findings more fully in chapter seven.[47]

In chapter eight of *De motu cordis*, Harvey does two important things: he describes the amount of blood passing from the veins through the heart and into the arterial vasculature and then characterizes the circular movement of the blood.[48] He begins this chapter expressing the fear that, "I may suffer the ill-will of a few, but dread lest all men turn against me." He is acutely aware of the magnitude of these claims, but also knows that his observations are irrefutable and hopes that the truth will win out. He proclaims, "The die has been cast."

Firstly, he determined the volume of blood passing through the heart in a given period of time and compares this volume with the amount of "juices" that come from the intestines over the same time. It was evident that the liver cannot produce enough blood to account for this volume of blood. The blood has to circulate and re-circulate in order to explain the volume of blood that moves through the heart in any given time. Further, he states:

> I subsequently verified, finding that the pulsation (contraction) of the left ventricle of the heart forces the blood out of it and propels it though the arteries into all parts of the body's system in exactly the same way as the pulsation of the right ventricle forces the blood out of that chamber and propels it through the artery-like vein into the lungs; finding further, that the blood flows back again through the veins and the vena cava and right up to the right auricle in exactly the same way as it flows back from the lungs through the so-called vein-like artery to the left ventricle .[49]

In this paragraph is contained the essence of what some consider the greatest medical discovery of all time—as earth shaking as Copernicus' heliocentric theory of the Solar System. Harvey had not only demonstrated the true physiology of the circulatory system, but had also verified the necessity of experimental observation. Such observations could and would destroy two millennia of errors. Medicine, indeed all of science, was now put on a totally different footing. The scientific world had been turned upside down. Simple authority, no matter how venerated, could not withstand the evidence of the senses. In the past, the philosophers had maintained the primacy of reason. Plato had made reason regal and the senses secondary; now this hierarchy had been inverted. Statistics was only beginning at this time.[50] Technology was limited and so, too, was the sophistication of observation and the experimental method. What Hippocrates and Galen had considered observation, experimentation, and experience seem now only child's play.

True science had just begun to sprout; it had much growth and maturation to achieve before it could be considered a mature science. The pace was slow and it was a stuttering start.

In spite of Harvey's impact on future medicine, he was at heart an Aristotelian. He began his lectures with some philosophical musings and viewed the heart, like the Sun, as the source of bodily heat. The Sun provided heat for the macrocosm and the heart for the microcosm.[51]

Robert Fludd

Robert Fludd (1574-1637 C.E.) was born at Shropshire, near Kent, of gentle, but not noble parents (though his father Thomas, who had been in the employ of Elizabeth I, was ultimately knighted).[52] Robert entered St. John's College, Oxford, in 1592. He was a serious, scholarly student, completing his B.A. in 1596 and M.A. in 1598. Developing an interest in astrology very early on, this was to guide much of his life and work. He also showed an interest in the occult arts. There were both Aristotelian and Platonic influences active at Oxford in the late sixteenth century and Robert gravitated toward Neo-Platonism. He was very religious and cultivated theological interests while at Oxford. St. John's was one of the Oxford colleges that had a medical fellow in residence and he may have fostered Fludd's medical interests. Following his M.A., as was the custom, he expanded his education by traveling abroad for six years in continental Europe. While wintering in Avignon, he wrote treatises on geometry, motion and astrology, as well as music and the art of memory. Additionally, he tutored several young noblemen in mathematics during this time.

Returning to England, he entered Christ Church College, Oxford, in 1604 and the following year received his M.B., M.D., and was licensed to practice medicine. He set up a practice in London and applied for admission to the Royal College of Physicians. Apparently this application to the College was punctuated by a series of exchanges between the "censor" of the college (who determined the qualifications of candidates) over the views Fludd held on Paracelsus and Galen, the later still the standard authority on medicine during the Elizabethan period. He was finally admitted in 1609. It was through the college that he met William Harvey. During these early years, he wrote a treatise on medicine, *Medicina Catholica* (Universal Medicine). Although he was familiar with the alchemical writings of Paracelsus, apparently he practiced primarily Galenic medicine.

Robert Fludd is of interest in the context of this book because he was a bright, well-educated physician of the early Enlightenment who straddled the fence between old and new medicine. A friend and supporter of Harvey's physiological findings, he still persisted in the ancient, centuries-old medicine that was to die a slow death over the next 200 years.[53]

It is instructive to look at Fludd's theory of health and disease in order to understand the extent to which Galenic theory penetrated the minds of some of the most learned physicians of the time. Galen's hold on medicine was strong, indeed, and not to be easily loosened. Many of the doctors of this period, though in the middle of a medical revolution, were largely unaware and unaffected by the changes at hand.

Fludd believed that disease was caused by a "wind" controlled by an "evil spirit" that excites the air. This tainted air could enter the body either through pores in the skin or the lungs and if there is a "weakness" in the bonds that hold the four humors in balance, disease will result.[54] The "air" spoken of here dates to the Hippocratic treatise on *Air, Water, Places*, which is echoed in Aristotle's *Meteorology*, both of which emphasize the impact of weather, climate and environment on disease induction. In the case of Hippocrates and Aristotle, there is less astrology and more astronomy (meteorology) underlying their ideas. For Fludd, however, astrology plays a central role in his theory.[55] The "weaknesses" spoken of include improper diet, lack of exercise, geography and the position of the planets. Fludd also experimented with alchemy, the last influenced by Paracelsus.

As covered before, Pythagoras had first developed the concept of microcosm and macrocosm. The microcosm (the individual human) was reflected in and influenced by the macrocosm (the heavens). This was detailed in Plato's *Timaeus* and played a pivotal role in the subsequent astrology of medicine, including Fludd's system of medicine.[56] He was a follower not only of Paracelsus, but also the Rosicrucians a mystical brotherhood with links to Hermes Trismagistus, Cabalism, and simple magic. It was in these obscure teachings that one was to decipher the mysteries of Nature. Fludd included the invisible fire of both Zoroaster and Heraclitus as well as the atomism of Democritus in his mystical medicine. The divine, as part of the macrocosm, was connected to the microcosm and the celestial forces that influenced health and disease. He also believed that as God had placed the Sun in the Solar System to provide heat, so too, the fire of the Sun was in the heart, and this provided the heat that warmed the blood and body, as Galen had proposed. In these concepts, Fludd displays his earnest religiosity. In terms of day-to-day medicine, Fludd, in following Galen, utilized uroscopy, along with astrology, in diagnosis.[57] He was taken with the therapeutic efficacy of wheat and wrote a treatise on this grain. He also believed in therapy at a distance.[58] One such treatment involved a "weapon-salve." If a patient had been injured by a knife, for example, the wound could be healed by applying the "weapon-salve" to the offending knife, thus heal the wound, even if the patient was far removed from the inciting instrument. Treatments of this type were based on the observation of effects "at-a-distance" displayed by magnets and amber. The Sun's rays acted at-a-distance, which also supported this view. Using urine from a patient and applying salves to weapons made it possible for the physician to diagnose and treat without ever seeing the patient and still collect a fee for services rendered.

In a treatise written by Fludd after Harvey published *De motu cordis* (1628), he appears to have been the first to support Harvey's theory of circulation, as mentioned earlier.[59] Such were the vagaries of the early Enlightenment.

Thomas Burnet

Another example of resistance to change is found in a book first published in 1685 by Thomas Burnet, who was physician to Charles II of England and several monarchs after him. His book, *Hippocrates Contractus*, (A Synopsis of Hippocrates) was a Latin translation of the original Greek Hippocratic Corpus.[60] The fact that a second edition was published in 1743, speaks to the hold Hippocrates and Galen had on English medical practitioners.[61] Abbreviated manuals of ancient authorities were favorite pocket references used by physicians of this period. Burnet wished to make the whole of the Corpus easily available "not only for beginners but it can also be [helpful] for the most versatile practitioner."[62] In the forward to his work, Burnet defends Hippocrates against the claims by Macrobius, in his *Commentary on the Dream of Scipio*, that Hippocrates had been, "unknowingly mistaken in his writings."[63] He denies Macrobius' assertion and calls Hippocrates "divinely inspired" and having been "the greatest philosopher [and] also the greatest physician (*summum suisse Philosophum, summum item Medicum*); a man with the greatest gift who will be praised always and everywhere." Further, he calls him, "a keen man of genius." Burnet notes that the governor of the Edinburgh Royal College of Physicians (of which Burnet was a fellow) thoroughly approved of his *Contractus*. It was also true that the royal College of Physicians of London affirmed these medical views. This included William Harvey who retained elements of Galenism in his practice.[64] Galenic medicine continued to be practiced into the nineteenth century. George Washington was treated by bloodletting the day before his death in 1799.[65]

The Royal Society of London was organized in 1662. Scientists, the likes of Robert Boyle, Robert Hooke, Edmond Halley and Isaac Newton, were among its most notable members and represented the cutting edge of the modern scientific revolution. These men were in large part responsible for the shifting scientific paradigm that was slowly permeating all of science including medicine. However, the persistent popularity of Hippocrates as attested to by Burnet's manual, gives evidence that it is hard to shed old beliefs and habits.

The Statistical Method

Modern science is not possible without statistics. Collecting data is necessary to making sense out of our world. Casual observation of nature can only give us a superficial view of our surroundings—an impression that may or may not be valid. There is no certitude in such observations. Much of what passed for "experience" in ancient Greece was nothing more than anecdotal data based on insufficient observations that could provide no certitude. What conclusions followed from these data were often no more than "opinion." Oftentimes what Descartes believed was "clear and distinct" truth turned out to be merely an intellectual mirage. Measurements of natural phenomena help define the various classes of objects found in nature but this is not enough to be called science:

> Measurements require some common understanding of their accuracy, some way of measuring and expressing the uncertainty in their values and the inferential statements derived from them.[66]

In other words, one can collect data and make comparisons with other data but it is necessary to have some way of telling whether the conclusions derived from these comparisons are certain or valid, allowing the conclusions to be useful in predicting future events. If the degree of uncertainty is too great, then the conclusions arrived at will be wrong often enough so that making useful predictions of future events and planning for appropriate future actions are useless. If experiments are set up so that they will not yield statistically valid results, then there is no purpose in making the observations. They will have no utility.

John Graunt (1620-1674 C.E.) was the first person to write a book on statistics *Natural and Political Observations on the Bills of Mortality in 1662.*[67] This had to do with mortality figures in London. The study was carried out in response to intermittent bubonic plague in London. The King wanted a population estimate and Graunt did this by using sampling techniques that included just three London parishes, extrapolating his findings to give an estimate of the total city population. This had never been done before. Somewhat later, Jacques Bernoulli (1654-1705) in *The Art of Conjecture* carried out the first probability studies showing that the greater the number of experiments, the closer the results come to predicted estimates, such as tosses of a die. For example, the prediction is that six will come up one-sixth of the time. The more tosses, the closer would be the observed occurrences of six to this predicted value. Abraham de Moivre (1667-1754) was the first to mathematically describe the normal biological, bell-shaped curve. Adolphe Quetelet (1796-1874) later used this to study the distribution of various human characteristics. William Playfair (1759-1823) introduced the line graph, bar graph and pie chart. John Snow (1813-1858), during the cholera epidemic of 1854, studied the geography of London's water supply and mortality pattern and found that a very high proportion of cases could be traced to one well. He found a sewer pipe within feet of the well that was contaminating it with *Vibrio comma*, the organism that causes cholera. Florence Nightingale (1820-1919) used statistics to support her campaign for hospital reform in England in the late nineteenth century. Many other advances in statistics have come about in the nineteenth and twentieth centuries.[68] Today the "bell-shaped" curves, standard deviation, p value, double-blind, crossover studies with matched controls are all commonplace statistical methods used in medicine. None of these techniques was available to the ancient or medieval physician. A p value of 0.05 (confidence that 95 percent of the time these same results will be obtained on subsequent trials) was not possible before the arrival of statistics. Without such techniques, however, one could not say with any confidence that St. John's Wort does or does not help depression.[69] Even with statistics, claims are made that turn out later to be erroneous but without this mathematical science modern medicine would be impossible.

Eighteenth-Century Medicine

Although the seventeenth century hosted the beginning of modern medicine, the eighteenth century demonstrated continuing medical progress. The subspecialties, as we know them today—psychiatry, surgery and obstetrics—began during this century.[70]

Aristotle had largely been toppled from his pedestal and a mad rush was on to find a new theoretical basis for medicine. One theory was championed by George Stahl (1660-1734). Stahl is best known for the phlogiston theory of combustion, which maintained that there was a principle or substance he named phlogiston, released when objects burned. Phlogiston was never found and oxygen was discovered later as a better explanation for combustion. In addition, Stahl postulated a vital principle that accounted for life itself. He resurrected the ancient idea of animism, which posited a vital force that inhabited all living things.[71] This was a metaphysical theory similar to ancient, even primitive ideas of life, but Stahl saw it as consistent with his theory of combustion, since phlogiston was also a kind of "spirit" that inhabited flammable materials. Vitalism is thought by some to be an offshoot of Lutheran spiritualism. More will be said about the Reformation later.

William Cullen (1710-1790) proposed "nervous energy" as the basis for health and disease. Cullen's followers classified all diseases as "sthenic" or "asthenic"— recommending either bleeding or purging, depending on which class a disease fell into.[72]

In addition to these vitalistic theories, there were the iatrochemists, following in the footsteps of Paracelsus. The use of metals and minerals was gaining favor in the medical community and began to replace herbal therapy, though the latter maintains its hold on medicine even today.[73] Arsenic and mercury were especially popular, though both undoubtedly produced more deaths than cures.[74] Another theory of medicine current in the eighteenth century was iatromechanics. This system was based on the philosophy of Rene Descartes.[75] He believed all matter was contiguous. A force applied to one part of the Universe was to be felt in all other parts. There was no empty space between bits of matter—no void or vacuum—as the Atomists had claimed. It was the "billiard ball" model later popularized by Pierre-Simon LaPlace (1749-1827).[75] This mechanistic model maintained that bodily function in health and disease was a matter of motion—the environment impacting the senses, which in turn influenced the inner workings of the body etc. Healthy food, activity and mental exercises made the body healthy. Unhealthy food, activity or thoughts caused disease.

Hermann Boerhaave (1668-1738) was not a theorist but rather a great clinician and lecturer. He introduced the clinico-pathological conference, which for the first time correlated clinical and pathological findings, as a teaching tool.[76] This was a major step forward in medicine. It was through such clinical advances that medicine gradually moved into the modern era.

The "empirical fever" that took hold in Britain, America and the Continent during the Enlightenment gradually crystallized into a truly scientific mode of medicine. It wasn't until the nineteenth century that technology made empirical, statistically valid medicine possible. An early example of this was the invention of the stethoscope by Rene Laënnec (1781-1826) in 1816.[77] After inventing the stethoscope, he studied 3,000 patients over the next three years, many of whom he was able to autopsy. This provided clinico-pathological correlations after their deaths, thus matching stethoscopic, antemortem findings with patho-physiological causes of these findings. This may have been the first truly modern clinical study and led the way to a medicine based on empiricism and not just anecdotal observations and speculative reasoning.

Notes

1.   Porter, R. 1997. *The Greatest Benefit to Mankind*, p. 201.
2.   Celsus was a first-century Roman medical writer.
3.   Celsus 1989, *De Medicina*, trans. W. G. Spencer, Loeb Classics (Cambridge, MA: Harvard University Press).
4.   Paracelsus 1983, *Hermetic Astronomy* (Edmonds, WA: Sure Fire Press). Hermes Trismagistus (thrice great Hermes) was a mysterious character dating to the time of the ancient Egyptians (as the god Thoth, Hermes for the Greeks). In fact, he was probably invented in the first century c.e. Many secrets of medical practice were attributed to him and Paracelsus drew inspiration from these "Hermetic Writings."
5.   Porter, R. 1997. *The Greatest Benefit to Mankind*, p. 201.
6.   Ibid., p. 202.
7.   Ibid., p. 203.
8.   An acute disease of the skin and subcutaneous tissue caused by a species of hemolytic streptococcus and marked by localized inflammation and fever.
9.   Any of various sulfates of metals, such as ferrous, zinc or copper sulfate.
10.   Mercury, arsenic and lead may cause serious consequences if used in high doses or over long periods.
11.   Paracelsus. 1999. *Essential Readings*, p. 50.
12.   Ibid., p. 49.
13.   Ibid.
14.   Sulfur and mercury certainly can be tested for but "salt" is a generic term and there are many salts that can be assayed.

15. Porter, R. 1997. *The Greatest Benefit to Mankind*, p. 204.
16. In this opinion, he was not far from the truth, in that uric acid, an irritating, needle-like crystal, is deposited in the affected joint causing the inflammatory reaction responsible for gouty arthritis.
17. Hippocrates. 1972, *Air, Water, Places.*
18. Aristotle. 1984, Meteorology.
19. Thompson, K.H. and Orvig, C. 2003, "The Boon and Bane of Metal Ions in Medicine," *Science*, 300:936-939.
20. Best, M. R. and Brightman, F. H. 1999. *The Book of Secrets of Albertus Magnus* (York Beach, ME: Samuel Weiser).
21. Christianson, J. 2006, Personal Communication.
22. Porter, R. 1997. *The Greatest Benefit to Mankind*, p. 179.
23. A device used for hanging a person until dead; a gallows.
24. Edelstein, L. 1943, "Andreas Vesalius: The Humanist," *Bulletin of the History of Medicine*, 14:547-561.
25. Singer, C. quoted in Nuland, S.W. 1989, *Doctors: The Biography of Medicine* (New York: Vintage Books), pp. 63-64.
26. Porter, R. 1997. *The Greatest Benefit to Mankind*, p. 180.
27. A plexus of veins at the base of the brain.
28. Porter, R. 1997. *The Greatest Benefit to Mankind*, p. 179.
29. Temkin, O, 1973, *Galenism: Rise and Decline of a Medical Philosophy* (Ithaca, NY: Cornell University Press), p. 14. One anecdote has it that Galen demonstrated the function of the recurrent laryngeal nerve in a squealing pig which was unable to make another sound as soon as Galen cut this nerve; all this carried out before a large audience of awestruck onlookers, doctors and lay people alike.
30. Ibid., p. 4.
31. Ibid., p. 141.
32. Nutton, V. 1996, *Cambridge Illustrated History of Medicine*, ed. R. Porter (New York: Cambridge University Press), p. 60.
33. Harvey, W. 1977, *The Circulation of the Blood*, trans. K. J. Franklin (New York: Dutton), p. v.
34. Ibid., p. viii.
35. Ibid., p. ix.
36. Porter, R. 1997. *The Greatest Benefit to Mankind*, p. 211.
37. *Pneuma* had a variety of meanings for the Ancients and Medievals. Most often, it was a kind of metaphysical substance that acted as a vital force. For some, *pneuma* was from the superlunary regions and emanated from the stars, thus, providing a measure of the divine mixed with the purely human aspects of earthly beings.
38. Hippocrates 1978, *Hippocratic Writings, The Regime for Health*, trans. J. Chadwick and W. N. Mann (New York: Penguin).
39. Porter, R. 1997. *The Greatest Benefit to Mankind*, p. 212.
40. Harvey, W. 1977. *On the Motion*, p. 13. Actually, this is not so difficult to imagine, since the air inhaled via the bronchial tree also carries out the waste carbon dioxide, without difficulty, with every breath inhaled and exhaled. Of course, blood does not flow through the bronchi.
41. Ibid., p. 213.
42. Ibid., p. 44.
43. Ibid.
44. Ibid., p. 45.
45. The portal vein drains the intestines, flows to the liver where it is broken up into many smaller veins, reassembled into the hepatic vein and then flows into the vena cava. Galen had the vena cava arising from the liver rather than the femoral

veins, which drain the legs. The renal veins also flow into the vena cava distal to the hepatic vein.
46. Ibid., p. 53.
47. Ibid., pp. 51-56.
48. Ibid., pp. 57-60.
49. Ibid., p. 58.
50. TimeWeb, 2005, Statisticians through History, http://www.bized.ac.uk/timeweb/reference/statisticians.htm.
51. Christianson, J. 2006, Personal Communication.
52. Fludd, R. 2001, *Robert Fludd*, ed. W. Huffman (Berkeley, CA: North Atlantic Books) pp. 15-17.
53. Debus, A.G. 1970. "Harvey and Fludd: The Irrational Factor in the Rational Science of the Seventeenth Century." *Journal of the History of Biology*, 3, 81.
54. Fludd, R. 2001. *Robert Fludd*, p. 18.
55. Dick, H. G. 1946, "Students of Physik and Astrology," *Bulletin of the History of Medicine and Allied Sciences*, 1:300-315.
56. Debus, A.G. 1970. "Harvey and Fludd."
57. Fludd, R. 2001. *Robert Fludd*, p. 33.
58. Ibid., p. 34.
59. Debus, A.G. 1970. "Harvey and Fludd."
60. Burnet, T. 1685, *Hippocrates Contractus, Approbation*, 1st Edition (Edinburgh: J. Reid).
61. Burnet, T. 1743, *Hippocrates Contractus*, 2nd Edition (London, Car. Davis & John Whiston, Fleetstreet).
62. Burnet, T. 1685, *Approbation*. All translations of the text are by the author, 2006.
63. Ibid., Preface.
64. Woolley, B. 2005. *Heal Thyself*, p. 184.
65. Crawl, T. 2000, "Bloodletting," *History Magazine*, Oct/Nov, pp. 15-17.
66. Stigler, S.M. 1986, *The History of Statistics: The Measurement of Uncertainty before 1900* (Cambridge, MA: Belknap Press of Harvard University Press), p. 1.
67. TimeWeb, 2006, "Statisticians through History," http://www.bized.ac.uk/timeweb/reference/statisticians.html.
68. Stigler, S. M. 1999, Statistics on the Table: The History of Statistical Concepts and Methods (Cambridge, MA: Harvard University Press).
69. Some twenty studies suggest that St. John's Wort has an anti-depressant effect about 1/20th that of Prozac.
70. Steensma, D. 2005. "Eighteenth Century Medicine: Enlightenment, Dogmatism, and Charlatanism," Mayo Clinic presentation, Feb. 24, 2005.
71. Ibid.
72. Ibid.
73. Crellin, J.K. and Philpott, J. 1989, *A Reference Guide to Medicinal Plants: Herbal Medicine Past and Present* (Durham, NC: Duke University Press).
74. Thompson, K.H. and Orvig, C. 2003. "Boon and Bane."
75. Strathern, P. 2000, *Mendeleyev's Dream: The Quest for the Elements* (New York: St. Martin's Press), p. 138.
76. Coulston, C. 1997, *Pierre-Simon LaPlace 1749-1827: A Life in Exact Science* (Princeton, NJ: Princeton University Press), p. 172.
77. Ibid.
78. Peak, L. 2004, "The Stethoscope," *History Magazine,* June/July, pp. 31-32.

Part 4

The Psychology of Change

8

Why the Delay?

There is no one reason why it took so long to structure and accept the modern paradigm of medical care. The roots of modern medicine's delayed growth are to be found in ancient Greece, Roman hegemony, the collapse of Rome along with its infrastructure, subsequent anarchy and the rise of the Western Church with its highly structured theology, among other factors. An attempt will be made in this final section to analyze these factors and the role each played in limiting and retarding change in our understanding and delivery of health care.

Greek Logic and Authority

Rational Greek medicine rose out of the ashes of ancient superstition and myth. Attempts by early civilizations to comprehend the mysterious and frightening world around them are understandable. It is not surprising that persistent, unproven but strongly held ideas about the world are found in every part of the globe and in every culture. These concepts are based on our inability to fully grasp the nature of the world and the insecurity associated with this uncertainty. Science doesn't have all the answers. Philosophy and religion try to fill in these gaps. Some tenaciously held (though errant) tenets are linked to prejudice, anxiety, tradition, emotions, egoism, monetary and/or political rewards. Much may be lost when change occurs. Change is a high stakes game.

The Greeks were among the first to move from superstition to science. However, their concept of science, including medicine, was not precise. Theirs was an embryonic concept of science. Hippocrates and his school began by throwing off the chains of superstition that bound them to folk medicine. In his treatise on the *Sacred Disease* (epilepsy) he says:

I do not believe that the so-called "Sacred Disease" is anymore divine or sacred than any other disease. It has its own specific nature and cause, but because it is completely different from other diseases men through their inexperience and wonder at its peculiar symptoms have believed it to be of divine origin.[1]

Hippocrates eliminates the possibility of disease as caused by the gods or any other supernatural source—disease is caused by the forces of Nature. All diseases have a rational basis.[2]

Hippocrates believed that "experience" in the practice of medicine was paramount. Medicine could not be learned quickly.[3] It took time to gain the experience necessary to the practice of good medicine. The experienced practitioner must, of course, be logical and rational in the interpretation of his experience but Hippocrates abhorred what he called "hypotheses" in understanding medicine. There were three schools of thought in medicine at the time: the Empiricists, Methodists, and Dogmatists. The Empiricists emphasized "experience" or observation of the patient. There was an element of skepticism in Hippocrates' empiricism, in that medicine was considered to be so complex that each patient needed to be dealt with on a completely individual basis. They maintained that there couldn't possibly be any rigidly dogmatic tenets that apply to all patients even if symptoms are essentially the same.[4] There are so many features associated with a given patient's disease at the moment a physician sees him or her that to apply a single set of rules for diagnosis, treatment or prognosis is impossible. The healer can only draw on his "experience" from past patients and situations to provide the best medicine at that moment. Things change for the patient from hour to hour and day to day and these variations must be accounted for. General medical knowledge or definitions are not possible for the Empiricist. Only particulars are valid. Age, gender, diet, exercise, geography, season of the year, ambient winds, critical days,[5] phase of the Moon, position of the planets, etc. must all be accounted for in treating the individual patient.[6]

The Methodist School relied on "experience" and observation of the patient but in a very limited way.[7] The Methodists did not believe it was necessary to know what part of the body was afflicted or its etiology. Age, constitution or habits of the patient were of no concern to the doctor. Climate and geography apparently did matter to the Methodist, however. There were only three diseases for the Methodist and these always involved the whole body: dry, fluid, and mixed. These states were determined by observation of the patient or his/her "natural excretions"—presumably urine, feces, phlegm, sweat, and so forth. Treatment is aimed at wetting the dry and drying the wet patient.[8] Theirs was a very simple scheme of diagnosis and therapy.

The Dogmatists were empiricists in the sense that they relied on "experience" and observation but, in addition, there was a strong philosophical element in their system. In contrast to the Empiricists, they espoused general theories and definitions of disease and therapy, which could be applied in diagnosing and treating the individual patient. The Empiricists did not believe "hidden" things were knowable in any sense. Hidden things were factors in diseases that could not be directly observed. Not so for the Dogmatists. They retained the rational, speculative aspect of Greek philosophy and were given to "logical" speculation about the unseen aspects of human disease. In other words, they could make up explanations for any disease, if these seemed rational or logical to the practitioner, even if unobserved.

The Greek physician appears to have made progress in the understanding of disease etiology, diagnosis and treatment in that they relied on observation of the patient as the primary and necessary part of medicine. However, their approach, though empirical in the broadest sense of this term, is still far from scientific medicine as practiced today. There were essentially no clinico-pathological correlations attempted except in some of the anatomical studies done later by the Alexandrians, Herophilus (c. 330-260 B.C.E.) and Erasistratus (c. 330-255 B.C.E.), who dissected human cadavers as noted earlier.[9] Though the Greeks had made a beginning, it could hardly be said that theirs was a lasting and productive influence on the road to modern medicine. These approaches seemed to the Greeks logical and internally consistent. In the absence of any better system, theirs remained the standard approach sustained by the unquestioned authority of the Ancients. The longer they were around, the greater their credibility. Like an old wine, they seemed more palatable with each passing year.

Roman Hegemony

The Romans brought stability to the Western World. The emperors, beginning with Augustus Caesar (reigned 27 B.C.E.- 14 C.E.), maintained relative peace throughout the empire. Pax Romana, spanning two hundred years, fostered a great deal of medical and other scientific writing.

Pliny the Elder

Pliny the Elder's (23-79 C.E.) *Natural History* contains sections on both medicine and cosmology.[10] Pliny notes that the Greeks used the term *cosmos* for the Universe, meaning 'ornament'—something of beauty—whereas the Latins labeled it *mundi*, that is, something with perfection and consummate grace.[11] This was a poetic view of the Universe but offered little information about the makeup of our world. As with much of Pliny's *Natural History,* his cosmology follows the Greeks and is filled with misinformation:

> The Sun, the ruler not only of the seasons and of the lands, but even of the stars themselves and the sky, moves in the midst of the planets: the Sun is greatest in size and power.[12]

Pliny is a geocentrist—the Sun moves, as do the planets, around the Earth and gives light to all the stars.[13] It is now known that the Sun is only a medium-sized star. Pliny also calls the Sun the soul or mind of the Universe. These concepts are patterned after Greek cosmology and help to reinforce the errors of the past.

Pliny presents a short herbal that follows the standard pharmacopeias inherited from the Greeks and other cultures before them. It contains the herbs passed down from ages past and provides many folk remedies, some of which are harmful. An example is the recommendation of *wormwood* for a variety of conditions including insomnia, intestinal "worms," soothing the bowels, nausea, flatulence, driving away gnats and, mixed with ink, as a method of preventing mice from eating the written word. It is even useful for dyeing the hair black.[14] If ingested, wormwood acts as a toxin to the brain and was banned from use in absinthe[15] early in the twentieth century because it caused dementia. Pliny was one of the authorities quoted well into the late Middle Ages. Seemingly the older the authority the more revered was their word. Pliny and other Romans were most influential in perpetuating the speculative theories of the Ancients. The Roman Empire was a symbol of authority and what was "Roman" automatically was surrounded by an aura of authenticity.

Authoritarianism

Galen, Ptolemy and, to a lesser extent, Celsus, Manilius, and Firmicus, were considered credible, if not sacrosanct authorities. Part of the reason for this reverence, it seems, was due to the authoritarianism originating in the imperial age of Rome and subsequently fostered by the Church after the Council of Nicaea, called by Constantine I, in 325 C.E. The Roman Empire had reached its pinnacle by the end of the first century C.E. Following Alexander the Great's conquests, his death and the beginning of the Hellenistic period, the stage was set for Rome to assume control over virtually all territories from the Middle East to the western reaches of the Mediterranean and north to southern Britain. They inherited the intellectual treasures of the Greeks and, utilizing their own military and engineering skills, built an infrastructure, remnants of which are still evident today, in their roads, buildings and aqueducts. With all this came power and authority unrivaled before or since. The Roman emperors adopted the *Theogony* of Hesiod (eighth century B.C.E.),[16] allowing them to claim divinity.[17] The power of the emperor and his empire were the ultimate authority—not to be questioned.

Born under the belly of this political behemoth was the fledgling Roman Catholic Church, which, within a few centuries, was to become a behemoth of another type. Its beginnings were Eastern, centered in the Levant. Initial growth was slow but by the time of Constantine I, it is estimated that up to 10 percent of the population in the East was Christian with a smaller percentage (~ 4 percent) in the West. Constantine was a shrewd ruler and knew that to maintain peace in the empire, factionalism could not exist within the Christian community. This belief may have been fostered in part by his ultimate victory over all other contenders for the imperial throne, culminating in his defeat of Maxentius at the Milvian Bridge. Legend has it that he attributed the victory to the Christian God, though this may have been an invention of his Christian biographer, Eusebius.[18] Whatever his motivations, Constantine realized the Eastern Church was developing an authority base—in some respects similar to his own—that would be useful in maintaining peace throughout the empire. Christians had been periodically persecuted over the first 250 years of their history. Seeing them as a help, rather than a hindrance to his goals, Constantine chose to make them allies instead of enemies. The emerging debate over the divinity of Jesus Christ was, however, proving to be a divisive issue, which he saw as impeding his peace plans. He called the Council at Nicaea (present-day Turkey) to settle the issue and restore harmony within the Church. Athanasius, bishop of Alexandria, held that Christ was co-eternal and consubstantial with God the Father. Arius, a presbyter, in Athanasius' diocese, believed Christ was created by God the Father, therefore, was neither co-eternal nor of the same essence as the Father.[19] Though there are limited scriptural bases for Athanasius' claim, he was able to persuade Constantine, who knew nothing of theology, that his was the "orthodox" view. The history of this debate is complex and whole books have been written on the subject of the Trinity. Suffice it to say, that Constantine ruled in favor of Athanasius, though he later reinstated Arius. After the Council, little changed theologically. In practice, the bishops who mostly sided with Arius continued preaching Arian views in their home dioceses. It was not until 381 that the Nicene

Creed finally won out.[20] Arianism, nonetheless, persisted for another 200 years in both the East and West.

Constantine fostered the growth of Christianity by granting favored tax status to "orthodox" Christians and by building a number of Christian churches. He did all this while allowing pagans religious freedom. Athanasius, after the Council of Nicaea, began a heavy-handed, at times violent, suppression of the Arians. This militant approach to orthodoxy was to persist to the time of the Reformation.

Authoritarianism was firmly established in the minds and hearts of Christians of the late Roman period. The Church willingly adopted a Roman style of control over its faithful. This approach suited its need to maintain orthodoxy and hegemony over its adherents. And when the Empire collapsed, the Church remained as the only institution capable of providing any semblance of order.

Heir to Rome: The Medieval Church

The Church had been largely a peaceful institution up to the time of Constantine.[21] However, he was a militant emperor. Claiming that God had been on his side at Milvian Bridge demanded a militant Christ—an image that had little, if any, scriptural support.[22] It was this "politicizing" of the Christian Church that appears to have provided the impetus for its mounting power and authority. The Vatican was to inherit the authoritarianism of the Roman Empire.

Though the Church initially had been largely eastern, events in the West promoted an increasing role for the Church in Rome. The Empire was beginning to crumble. Rome was repeatedly under threat. Seemingly, the only authority available to manage these crises was the Bishop of Rome. The government centers were decaying while great basilicas rose up in their stead. Although the Catholic Church maintains that there was an unbroken line of authority from Peter forward, the title of Pope was not used until after the fourth century. Pope Leo I (reigned 440-461) was instrumental in avoiding the sack of Rome in 452, when Attila the Hun left Rome unscathed. This may have been due to Attila's lack of resources but Leo took credit for saving the capital. Leo was the first strong bishop of Rome and in large part is responsible for making the papacy what it is today. As "heir to Peter," Leo was determined to establish his authority over other bishops of the West. He saw himself as the legal successor to Peter through an unbroken line of "legally" elected bishops reaching back to the first bishop of Rome, who may or may not been Peter. This concept of "apostolic succession" has been the warrant for papal and ecclesiastical authority ever since. A reminder of this chain of command is engraved on St. Peter's Basilica today, proclaiming that Peter is the rock upon which the Church's authority is based—authority given to Peter by Christ.

In his dealings with all other bishops, both eastern and western, Leo made it known that he was head of the Church. All heretics (those questioning his authority) were dealt with sternly. Civil authority was seen as tied to ecclesiastical hegemony—a connection lasting until the formation of the Italian state. In the 1860s, the Papal States were reduced to a small area adjacent to Rome—now a one-mile square area known as Vatican City.[23] Leo published a series of decrees dealing with church government, authority of bishops and ordination of clergy—all strengthening the Pope's authority. It was Leo's version of the two natures of Christ that was ultimately adopted as orthodoxy at the Council of Chalcedon in 451. He asserted his authority over all of the Christian Church, including the Eastern Church—a tenuous relationship at best and one that was not to last.[24] The bond, and later the battle between State and Church was to continue into the modern period. Pope versus emperor or king was a persistent theme. Justinian (483-565 C.E.) involved himself in theological maters including the nature of Christ. Medieval kings appointed their own bishops, ignoring the will of the Vatican, resulting in the "Investiture Controversy." The authoritarianism of the Church reached its peak during the reign of Julius II (reigned 1503-1513 C.E.), the "Warrior Pope," who personally led armies against Bologna and Venice (among others) in defense of the Papal States— the spiritual and corporeal worlds at odds as the soul and body of wo/man so often seem to be.[25]

The hegemony of the Roman Empire was inherited by the Church. Its authoritarianism, though not as militarily powerful, was spiritually equal in power to the former Roman Empire. It held sway over both the minds and bodies of the "faithful" in a manner heretofore unknown. Its system of rewards and punishments (Heaven, Hell, excommunication, and Inquisition) held the people in homage and bondage to the Church for centuries. What the Church held to be true on Earth was true in heaven. Any concept deemed harmful to the human soul (and Church authority) was rejected and this included modern ideas of science and medicine. The Catholic Church is one of the most conservative of institutions and change within it occurs at a snail's pace. The Galileo Affair is a classic case of ecclesiastical resistance to change. His views were not officially sanctioned until the nineteenth century.

Anxiety and Insecurity

With the collapse of the Western Empire in 476, life became more difficult for the common person and more combative for the nobleman. The Roman infrastructure gradually fell apart. Roads disintegrated and communication dwindled along with the roads. Water supplies became more fragile, as the aqueducts decayed. Hygiene lessened as sewage systems plugged up. Centralized government was replaced by sectional "warlords" who continually fought one another over control of land and its associated wealth. Society became agrarian; cities declined. After the death of Theoderic in 526, Justinian was intent on ridding the West of its Ostrogothic (and Arian) government. Rome, which had an estimated population of one million inhabitants at the time of Trajan (d. 117),[26] had shrunk to a mere 30,000 people as a result of warring and consequent disorder.[27] Much of Rome became pasture for cattle. By the end of the sixth century, eyewitnesses described crumbling buildings, aqueducts and sewers, collapsed granaries, and statues violated, The yellow Tiber carried dead cattle and often human remains. Many inhabitants of Rome were starving to death, others dying of pestilence. Malaria was endemic in the swampy Campagna. Those who could afford it fled to Constantinople. Others retreated to the relative comfort of the countryside. As it was in Rome, so it was in much of the West. The only hope seemed to lie with the spiritual comfort of the Church.

In 500 c.e., the people of Rome, stricken with plague, walked in procession, heads bowed, to the Mausoleum of Hadrian, where it is said:

> The Archangel Michael, captain of the heavenly host and guardian of the sick, appeared in the sky sheathing his sword as a sign that the plague would soon be over. [28]

Safety from material, mental and spiritual harm seemed only to come from religion. Local lords could offer only limited relief from the anguish of war and, little or none, from want and worry. Paul of Tarsus had described the Last Judgment as a "day of anger"[29] and Augustine attributed all human ills to Original Sin. Thus, the insecure life of the early Middle Ages, with its many sufferings and sorrows was to be blamed on the sins of the unrepentant. God was a wrathful Father in the Torah, a revengeful being raining down punishment on all who disobeyed Him.[30] This view of God suited the Christians of the Middle Ages. Their life was filled with fear and trepidation. The Church Fathers supported this portrait of the Deity.[31] Salvation was always in question and no one, no matter how good, was assured a place in heaven according to Augustine (and later Luther). Plato had seen the human psyche as at continual war with itself. Christians saw this as a battle with the devil and one could never relax. The inherent sinfulness of humankind was ever present. Death and damnation might come at any moment.

Besides the spiritual refuge of the Church, there was the material safety of her churches and monasteries. The high, thick walls still evident around Vatican City and many other medieval cities remind us of the constant threat posed by both internal and external enemies. Rothenburg, Germany, as one example, remains a walled city today. During the Middle Ages there were hundreds of convents and monasteries that provided security for many. The nobles had their castles and these offered refuge in times of war but the commoners could find respite from day to day anxieties only within the confines of religious houses. In the milieu of the Middle Ages, the Church and safe sanctuary went hand in hand. With this came a firm hold on men and women's intellectual lives, an intellectualism that became increasingly more restricted.

Karen Armstrong offers "fear" as a major motivating force in the belief systems of fundamentalists.[32] In her book, *Jerusalem*, she notes that security issues have played a major role in the history of Israel.[33] It may be that fear and insecurity have been building blocks of the foundations of all faiths for many centuries. As humans, we have a need to believe in something that makes us feel secure against the threats that seem to confront us on all sides. This demands a belief in something greater and more powerful than oneself. Belonging to such an institution empowers us and gives us a sense of community—a kind of social security, if you will. A Darwinian survival drive may underlie anxiety as part of natural selection. It preserves us along with the species as a whole.

We all are subject to wishful thinking because it helps us face the future. The idea of heaven allows us to look forward to something better in the "life hereafter."[34] When undergoing chemotherapy for a terminal cancer, it helps to think that the treatment will "cure" the cancer or at least prolong life. As long as we have hope for a better future, life seems worthwhile. These beliefs allay anxiety. It is more important for most of us to believe in myths, no matter how outlandish, than to give into uncertainty and despair. Belief in a medical system that offers little, if any, hope of cure is better than giving in to hopelessness. The same holds for prayer and religious ritual; they offer the possibility of relief from sorrow and suffering.

Anxiety and insecurity are the cement that holds us to governments, no matter how corrupt and theocracies, no matter how restrictive. Conservative institutions provide the most security in times of uncertainty. Liberal views are best accepted when one is comfortable and safe. Unsettled times are not times for change. These are the times we hang on to old ideas. Political unrest or even revolt may occur at these times but intellectual revolutions seldom do. This includes medical revolution.

Anti-Intellectualism

Early on, the Christian Church found it necessary to maintain tight reins on the religious tenets of its adherents. Pagels makes the point that "Apostolic Succession" has provided the basis for Church authority since Peter.[35] This direct line of authority has limited the hierarchy of the Church to a small number of men whose views are incontestable. In the early Roman Church, the bishop of Rome was elected by all local Christians—lay as well as religious. Later, however, the ordination of priests was in the hands of bishops who, in turn, were selected by church insiders, most of whom were interested in maintaining the status quo. As a result, the hierarchy has become increasingly more conservative. This is true of any long-standing institution. As an example, interpretation of the Bible has been limited to a few select theologians and, if any of these diverge from "orthodoxy" as defined by the Vatican they are subject to censorship. It is believed that only Catholic orthodoxy can provide salvation. The souls of a billion Catholics are at stake and they run the risk of eternal damnation if misled by the clergy. The hierarchy of the Church felt they were carrying a heavy burden and any means was justified, as long as it "saved" souls.

As we have seen, orthodox theology is sometimes politically based, and is not an empirical science, relying on ones interpretation of the Bible and "tradition." Thus it is often the product of contentious, speculative debate. As a result, religious dogma is frequently spurious and anti-intellectual. Politics, egoism, economics, biases and other factors may enter into the making of orthodoxy. As a result of all these non-theological considerations, blind acceptance of many elements of faith was frequently required. The authority of the hierarchy had to be unquestioned or political, economic and/or personal disasters might follow. The medieval Church had too much to lose, if their credibility were questioned.

Paul of Tarsus spoke Greek but had little knowledge of the philosophers of ancient Greece. He denounced "the empty logic of the philosophers."[36]

This view set the stage for the dogmatic tendencies found in the early Church. It was the word of Christ that was to be believed and nothing else. Even if an idea were supported by the senses, it must yield to this higher truth. Constantine assumed a similar stance when he asserted:

We have received from Divine Providence the supreme favor of being relieved from all error.

It was such convictions that allowed Constantine and later emperors, Justinian, as one example, to "pontificate" regarding all manner of topics with absolute impunity.

Christ was *logos*, the word made flesh. It was He who brought God the Father's word to the world. "The Word was God and the Word was with God" (John 1:1). *Logos* can be interpreted in a number of ways including as meaning "reason," "rational" or "master plan." However one views it, *logos* was the reasoning or pronouncements of God, incarnate. These dicta were not to be questioned. Later, John Chrysostom (d. 407 C.E.), a staunch supporter of Paul's view of truth, suggested that:

We restrain our own reasoning, and empty our mind of secular learning, in order to provide a mind swept clear for the reception of divine words.[37]

Basil, bishop of Caesarea, seconds this idea:

Let us Christians prefer the simplicity of our faith to the demonstrations of human reason.... For to spend much time on research about the essence of things would not serve the edification of the church.[38]

Many writers of the fourth and fifth centuries echo these views. In essence, there was nothing to be gained from scientific research. It would profit nothing in terms of the life hereafter. A certain Philastrius of Brescia went so far as to imply that the search for scientific knowledge was heresy, pure and simple. He asserted that to attribute earthquakes to "the very nature of the elements" rather than to "God's command" was heterodoxy. This anti-intellectual mindset led, increasingly, to less and less interest in the classics and more and more focus on scriptural and ecclesiastical readings. Simplicius of Cilicia (c. 530 C.E.) wrote several commentaries on Aristotle's works[39] but following the closing of the ancient philosophical schools in Athens by Justinian in 529 C.E., none of Aristotle's works was available in the West until the twelfth century. Some have suggested that the sacking of the Alexandrian Library was allowed by Bishop Theophilus because classical works were pagan, providing no spiritual value.[40] Virtually all Maya writings were burned for the same reason. Leo I is reported to have said that, "We uphold the

Nicene Creed but avoid difficult questions beyond human grasp. Clever theologians soon become heretics." Discussions and debates of all sorts dwindled as time went on. Isidore of Seville complained that books were hard to find when he compiled his *Etymologies.* The Venerable Bede's (672-735 C.E.) library consisted of commentaries on the scriptures, patristic treatises (Latin only) and such secular works as Pliny's *Natural History.* Secular knowledge, according to Augustine, was useful only insofar as it helped in biblical exegesis. For the illiterate of both East and West, only icons or religious art provided any learning. Plato continued to be studied because his writings seemed to lend themselves to Christian theology (if properly interpreted). By the twelfth century, his *Timaeus* was the only one of his works extant in the West. Many Greek writings, even if available, could not be read or translated into Latin. Ptolemy's *Almagest* is an example of this problem.

Galen's theory of anatomy and physiology was easily assimilated into a Christian context because he held that God had created each part of the human body for a specific purpose. His was a teleological system utilizing Aristotle's fourth (final) cause.[41] Galen was a pagan who, at one point, criticized Christians for not thinking rationally. This apparently did not put off Christian writers—Galen's works survived without criticism for 1,500 years. We have seen this kind of selective theology before. The Neo-Platonism of Augustine and others made it easy to slide over any embarrassing theological contradictions, in part, because the soul was more important than the body. Even if Galenic medicine had its deficiencies, all that really mattered was eternal salvation. Health of the body was secondary to spiritual health of the soul—one more example of the anti-intellectualism of the age. This anti-intellectual trend undoubtedly played a significant role in the persistence of medieval medicine, as well as, the slow pace of scientific progress in other fields. It is more comfortable sleeping with old ideas than exercising the intellect in pursuit of new knowledge. Such intellectual "couch potatoes" rest easily in their ignorance.

The Reformation

It is uncertain as to how influential Protestantism was in fostering or impeding scientific thought. Luther, more than most men, "hungered after" certitude.[42] The certainty he sought, however, was spiritual and not scientific. He found Copernicus' theory of the Solar System untenable. The Bible was the ultimate word on all things, both sacred and secular, and it was clear to Luther that Genesis (I:1) left no doubt as to how the world was made and how it worked. Luther believed firmly that the Earth was at the center of the Universe.[43] Philip Melanchthon (1497-1560) was of a like mind according to many authors but Kusukawa claims this is not entirely true.[44] He suggests that Melanchthon was more practical in his view of Copernicus. Melanchthon did say in a letter to a friend that Copernicus' heliocentric concept was "absurd."[45] However, Melanchthon was primarily concerned with moral rather than natural philosophy in this instance. What was important was getting humans into heaven, not how the heavens worked.[46]

Melanchthon believed fervently in astrology. Astrology and the beauties of astronomy were evidences of a providential God. Copernicus' masterful mathematical calculations provided the faithful with yet another way of knowing how marvelous the Deity was. Greater understanding of natural philosophy made moral philosophy all the more real and practical. The more accurately celestial positions could be determined, the better were astrological predictions and the greater our knowledge of God. Copernicus himself cast horoscopes and this fit well with Melanchthon's ideas. Copernicus could not be all bad, if he supported astrological tenets. Melanchthon chose to largely ignore the Polish canon's less savory ideas of heliocentrism and emphasize the glories of God's Universe.

The Reformation undoubtedly ushered in a new view of ancient authority. Luther, and those of like mind, thwarted the power of the Pope. Leo X (reigned 1513-1521) had initially minimized the threat Luther posed to Church authority. Leo was an affable, lovable man who liked to please people, spending much of the Vatican wealth on patronage of the arts. He ran the papal coffers dry but was committed to a makeover of St. Peter's Basilica. Indulgences were to pay for this and on the Ides of March 1517, he promulgated the indulgences that were to forever diminish papal authority. National sentiment soon stirred resentment and Frederick III, elector of Saxony, who opposed papal fiscal interference, set about to protect Luther and his ninety-five theses from the pope's wrath.[47] In due course, Leo realized the threat Luther posed to the Vatican and first Luther was ordered to respond to questions asked by Cardinal Cajetan at Augsburg. Then in 1520, Leo issued a bull condemning forty-one statements made by Luther, authorized burning of his books and gave him sixty days to recant his heretical views.[48] In September 1520, Leo issued a bull of excommunication that prompted Luther to publish his famous *The Babylonian Captivity of the Church*.[49] The die had been cast and the

Reformation snowballed throughout Europe. Papal authority had been broken by a little-known professor of scripture from Wittenberg.

How did this revolution affect the course of science and especially medicine? It certainly allowed dissenters to do so with some degree of impunity though there were many cases of death imposed by Protestants leaders on those they considered heretical. It was all a matter of geography and local politics. Undoubtedly the Reformation allowed more freedom of action for many scientists and doctors, though this freedom was not immediately felt by all "freethinkers" and conservative tendencies found in the various Protestant sects were often as restrictive as those in the Roman Church. Religious conservatism was quick to surface during the Reformation. It was evident in England during the seventeenth century with the Puritans and the mid-century civil war, as well as, Switzerland with Calvin and in Germany with Luther. The Counter-Reformation fired up the Inquisition to new levels of injustice in dealing with heterodoxy. All these forces constrained scientific thought for some time. Newton, who was a closet Unitarian, found it necessary to conceal his thoughts on the Trinity.[50] Thus, the Reformation probably had a mixed effect on science, loosening the hold of the Roman Church while spawning conservative thought that is evident in some of the issues we face in America today.

Egoism: The Need to be Right

Egoism plays a role in most belief systems. We all like to be "right." As we have seen, one reason we believe things that cannot be established as "scientifically true" relates to the force of authority.[51] It is evident that ancient writers influenced the views of later ages. Scripture and other holy writings provide the written foundations of spiritual authority for all religions. From its inception, Christianity utilized the collective authority of Church Fathers, just as the Greeks had relied on Hesiod, Homer, Plato, and Aristotle. Their antiquity, authority and logic endowed them with persistent credibility. Rationalism, especially as promoted by Plato and Aristotle, ruled the realm of truth for many centuries. The senses could not be trusted. As René Descartes put it in the seventeenth century, what is "clear and distinct" to the mind, must be true.[52] God is not a deceiver, Descartes claimed, so what was "clear and distinct" could not be false—God would not put errant ideas in the minds of men and women. Adherence to these authorities implies egoism. What we are taught by parents, teachers, friends, religious, or secular authorities, becomes part of our personal identity. These beliefs are necessary to ones sense of self and security. To abandon these foundations is to deny our very identity. It would make us "wrong" about our self and our world. Undercutting the concept of self is a potential personal disaster. It is too frightening for most of us to allow—ego strength dwindles and with it, confidence in the very underpinnings of our world. We become lonely and ill-equipped to deal with the "real" world in which we live. This is why we must be "right."[53] For many, absolutes make for certainty and certainty provides the security necessary for a comfortable life.

Whether we believe in reason, experimentation or both, trust rests on accepting some credible authority and the perceived merits of their arguments. The same applies to beliefs in myths, religions or cults. When we believed in Santa Claus or the Easter Bunny, it was because our parents told us they existed and we trusted our parents as credible authorities. If one believes in the tenets of the Church of Latter Day Saints, it is because John Smith said so in the Book of Mormons and we see him as credible. If one is Jewish, it is because s/he believes God enlightened Moses and the other prophets while inspiring the writing of the Torah and the rest of the Bible. The same holds for the New Testament of Christians. The followers of Jim Jones were willing to take cyanide on the authority of this charismatic leader.

It has been said that one person's myth is another person's religion. How many of the ancient Greek myths were accepted as true by the informed Greek is uncertain, nonetheless, these stories appear to have been well received by the average Greek.[54] Adults don't believe in Santa Clause; children do. Theists believe that God created the Universe in six days; Deists don't. Some religious groups believe in Creationism; some believe in Evolution. Many have a fervent belief in God; others (atheists) are strict materialists. Humanists may or may not believe in God but this concept is not necessary to their belief system.[55] It is evident that all these groups have some basis for their beliefs. The Creationists hold the Bible as absolute; the Evolutionists cite scientific evidence to support their views. How valid the one warrant is as compared to the other, is not the concern of this book. Rather, it is to analyze why we believe what we believe.

Whatever the reasons given for adherence to one belief system or another, they are usually deep-seated and tied intimately to our sense of self—to our ego. Ego strength is essential in coping with life. A strong ego makes living life easier and situational anxieties less burdensome. Daily stressors can be dealt with more easily and comfortably if we have a strong belief system to sustain us. A firmly held belief system is a kind of security blanket. Letting go of such a system and adopting another is too unsettling for most of us to readily accomplish. This is true for the highly educated as well as the less schooled. It makes no difference how smart or academically sophisticated one might be. More often than not, it is an arduous emotional journey to accept new concepts, especially ones that contradict previously strongly held beliefs. Reason plays a minor role in this process.

Egoism and emotions are usually evident in the rejection of any new idea. Acceptance of a new belief is also an emotional journey and involves willingness to restructure the image we have of our self and our world. This can be a very painful process.

The Clan Mentality

Belonging to a community provides survival potential for the individual and his/her society. [56] A "clan mentality" was the basis, presumably, for the formation of primitive societies. It promoted clan strength and improved the chances for survival of the clan. Anything that strengthens the community tends to be supported by its members. Loyalty to the community is paramount. Whatever sets the group apart from other groups, making it special, better or stronger, most clan members believe without critical proof. There is no evidence that personality traits vary from one culture to another.[57] In other words, fundamentally we differ little from people of other cultures. Nonetheless, each group sees itself as the chosen people—chosen by God. Our homeland is sacred and destined by God to be ours for all time. We have sacred spaces that are not to be defiled by non-believers—beliefs that many would be willing to die for. Ours is the one and only true religion, state and/or culture. Only our "faithful" will go to heaven—all infidels are condemned to hell. We are more powerful, diligent and intelligent than other peoples. The foreigner, barbarian, those of different skin color, religions and/or cultures are necessarily inferior and must be shunned or destroyed. All these attitudes help the community to prosper over other communities. Or at least this seemed the case before we became part of the global community. We feel more secure, less fearful and more content when our group is strong or perceived to be so. The community's individual and collective ego is strengthened, which makes for a better chance of clan (and species) survival. It is the confident army—God is on our side—that is most often victorious in battle.

Any belief that fosters community solidarity is accepted no matter how irrational. This is not to say that these beliefs are intrinsically bad. They certainly are functional and make for a more cohesive society. This mentality played a major role in medieval society. What society accepted was usually accepted by the individual. Divergence from these norms meant isolation from society as a whole, followed by insecurity and diminished ego strength. Though many privately questioned the medieval physician's credibility, when frightened enough, they returned to the time-honored therapies these healers provided.

Francis Bacon (1561-1626) tried to summarize the various types of unscientific thought in the *New Organon*.[58] Bacon defines four "Idols": that of the Tribe, the Cave, the Marketplace, and Theater. "The Idols of the Tribe have their foundations in human nature itself. Proper inductive reasoning is distorted by biases inherent in human nature. The clan mentality, the egocentricity of *homo sapiens* and our limited understanding of the Universe, all account for errors arising from our nature. The Idol of the Cave, like Plato's shadows on the cave wall, are distorted images of reality caused by each individual's biases based on prior life experiences, education, and circumstances. The Idol of the Marketplace is "formed by the intercourse and association of men with each other." We are influenced by those around us. Finally, the Idols of the Theater are derived from the dogmas and philosophies of those who have developed philosophical and theological systems in the past and are considered unassailable authorities. Each of these Idols is evident in our personal belief systems as well as in those of many groups that disagree with us. It is always easier to see errors and loose logic in others. Francis Bacon's Idols have been discussed in one form or another above. The influences of others—family, friends, associates; institutions, religions — the culture that shapes our mores, past and present, have all provided answers to unanswerable questions. Bacon's Idols are another way to understand the irrational side of human thought.

Bertrand Russell wrote an article in the 1920s explaining why he was not a Christian.[59] In the article, he very rationally explains his reasons for this decision and deftly dismisses the various arguments for the existence of God, He emphasizes the emotional factor in religious belief, naming "fear" as a major factor in the genesis of religion (as Armstrong also asserts). His arguments reflect some of the reasons given above for the popularity of religion. However, Russell's arguments, including those outlined earlier, in a real sense, miss the point. The reality of religion cannot be judged by rational standards. As Mary, Queen of Scots said, "I could not reason but I know what I must believe."[60] In the final analysis, religious belief is founded on faith and faith alone. This, likewise, is true for most of ones firmly held beliefs. Their reality is not rational; it is spiritual, psychological or mystical but not empirical. Beliefs cannot be "proven" but this does not diminish their reality. There is no one truth. There is always uncertainty. Truth for one is not truth for another. Abelard of Bath (c.1080-c.1137) put it best when he observed that for some, truth is in the head and for others, it is in the heart.[61] As Karen Armstrong has pointed out, the difference lies with the concepts of *logos* and *mythos*.[62] Each has its place in the inner world of the rational animal, as Thomas Aquinas defines humans. There is something here for the rational, as well as the animal in us all.

In the end, it would seem that the only thing that matters, when speaking of truth, is its utility. The laws of physics are 'real' because they have a certain internal consistency and practical value. We can make predictions about the world using these laws—predictions that "work" in our everyday life. In its simplest form, we know that if we jump out of a tall building, there is a high probability that this will be the end of life, as we know it. Physical laws can take us no further than this but they can help us stay out of harm's way and provide useful gadgets to make life easier and better. In a similar vein, the reality of religion and other belief systems is also utilitarian. Belief in various tenets can provide solace, cheer, and companionship in hard times. It gives us something to look forward to. Prayer, meditation, and ritual lower the blood pressure, raise skin temperature and increase endorphins—all comforting physiological responses. Religion also "works" in this sense and can make life better (though not always). The warrant for science is the belief in the scientific method, for religion, it is faith. Viewed from the scientific standpoint, faith appears baseless and science, as seen by the faithful, appears shallow. These same points can be applied to ancient and medieval medicine. Being treated, talked to, listened to, and attended to all have their beneficial effects. The placebo response comes into play but there is more to medical care than psychological support. Treatments sometimes actually help—more so today than in the past. Whether treatment be biologically effective or not, it may incur inexplicable benefits. Thus, ancient and medieval medicine, though largely ineffective and often harmful, provided hope for the patient and family. Why throw away the Galenic system when there is nothing better with which to replace it? If reason (*logos*), the spirit *mythos*) or preferably both are satisfied, the healer has achieved his/her goal. The patient feels better and is better.

Change

Change under any conditions is difficult, as we have seen.[63] It is easier to stay with the status quo. Even during crises that demand change, it is at best difficult. One has to deal with both the crisis and change. Change may entail a threat to life style, finances, control over one's life, loss of status and many more disruptions that are troublesome for all of us. It may impact the ego. Once having found the "truth" (as we see it), to abandon this "truth" and accept another is both intellectually and emotionally difficult. If once having settled on an "absolute" truth, it is even harder to change—if a truth is absolute, how can it be abandoned? Even Euclid's *Element*, once thought infallible in the realm of mathematics, has come under attack in the past two centuries.[64] How could such a standard system of mathematics be questioned? It is unthinkable.

Change comes hard, but beginning in the sixteenth century a new attitude emerged regarding innovation and re-examination of ancient dogma. Men and women came to believe that investigating the natural world, full of mysteries just waiting to be solved, was a worthy pursuit. Learned societies were established in Italy, France, and England. Literacy was on the rise and, of course, typeset had been invented by Guttenberg—the most significant invention of the Renaissance. The acquisition and dissemination of knowledge began to snowball. In the sixteenth century, the telescope, microscope, thermometer, barometer, the air pump (vacuum machine), and pendulum clock were all invented.[65] Many more innovations followed. At first, people laughed at scientific societies and their new fangled gadgets. But this soon passed and wonder replaced cynicism. Change, at least scientific change, was becoming commonplace and more easily assimilated by the general population. A mad rush in the sciences was forthcoming—medicine, chemistry, biology mathematics and physics were all on a fast track toward new ideas. This transformation inevitably led to a new medical paradigm. It was no longer the humors that were out of harmony within the body, but bacteria, chemicals, pressures, rhythms, temperatures, electrical circuitry, cell replication, and genes. Blood, bile and phlegm were still around but blood had too little hemoglobin, too much iron, too many or too few leukocytes. Bile was found to be of much less importance in health and phlegm was mainly a sign of disease rather than the cause of it. The lack of serotonin rather than excess black bile caused depression. Apoptosis[66] may account for aging rather than a cold, dry constitution. Herbs were largely replaced (but not entirely) by complex molecules made by bacteria, either naturally, like penicillin, or genetically engineered as with insulin and a host of other therapeutic wonders. Diseases now are due to molecular disturbances rather than disharmony in fluids and qualities of the body. All these changing concepts have not come easily. The process of change as we have seen comes at a cost. We must pay a heavy price in terms of emotional and physical toil and turmoil.

Notes

1. Hippocrates. 1978. *Hippocratic Writings*, p. 237.
2. Longrigg, J. 1993, *Greek Rational Medicine:* Philosophy and Medicine from Alcmaeon to the *Alexandrians* (New York: Routledge) p. 1.
3. Edelstein, L. 1967. *Ancient Medicine*, p. 190.
4. Ibid., pp.199-200.
5. Fevers, that is, diseases characterized by fever, were believed to follow a certain course related to the pattern of the fever. Certain clinical changes can be expected on certain days. Recovery, relapse or even death is expected to occur on these critical days.
6. There developed a later 'Hellenistic' Empiricism, which incorporated some philosophical or speculative elements (hypothesis) into their approach to medicine but continued to rely heavily on observation of the patient.
7. Ibid., pp. 179-184.
8. Curiously, this is still a maxim in treating skin diseases.
9. Porter, R. 1997. *The Greatest Benefit to Mankind*, p. 66.
10. Pliny. 1991. *Natural History*, pp. 10-41, 224-267.
11. Ibid., ,p. 11.
12. Ibid.
13. It was commonly held that the Sun lighted all the stars as well as the Moon. "He (the Sun) lends his light to the rest of the stars," according to Pliny.
14. Ibid., p. 249.
15. Absinthe was a licorice flavored alcoholic beverage popular in the late nineteenth century in America and Europe.
16. Hesiod. 1983. *Theogony and Works and Days*, trans. M. L. West (Oxford: Oxford University Press).
17. Freeman, C. 2002. *The Closing of the Western Mind*, p. 48.
18. Ibid., p. 157.
19. Ibid., p. 164.
20. The Emperor Theodosius rigged the Council of Constantinople (381) so that the theology of the Trinity was firmly established in the form proclaimed at the Council of Nicaea.
21. Early on there had been violence associated with the election of the Bishop of Rome.
22. In Revelations (19: i.1-16), there is a warrior of heaven on a white horse with a sharp sword, who is sent down to destroy the pagans. It is not at all clear that this was Christ. Such an image was certainly at odds with Christ's Sermon on the Mount.

23. Duggan, C. 1994. *A Concise History of Italy* (Cambridge: Cambridge University Press), p. 138.
24. The formal split of East and West came in 1054.
25. Durant, W. 1955. *The Renaissance: A History of Civilization in Italy from 1304-1576 A.D.* (New York: Simon & Schuster), pp. 441-447.
26. Hibbert, C. 1995. *Rome: The Biography of a City* (New York: Penguin), p. 53.
27. Ibid., p. 74.
28. Ibid., p. 75.
29. Freeman, C. 2002., p. 305.
30. Armstrong, K. 1993, *A History of God: The 4,000 Year Quest of Judaism, Christianity and Islam* (New York: Ballantine Books) pp. 276-277. This is the type of god Luther believed in and is the god of many today.
31. Freeman, C. 2002. *The Closing of the Western Mind*, p. 305.
32. Armstrong, K. 2000. *The Battle for God* (New York: HarperCollins).
34. Cahane, H., & Cavender, N. 1998. *Logic and Contemporary Rhetoric: The Use of Reason in Everyday Life* (New York: Wadsworth), pp. 116-117.
35. Pagels, E. 1979. *The Gnostic Gospels* (New York: Vintage Books), pp. 10-11.
36. Op. cit. Freeman, C. 2002, p. xviii.
37. Ibid., p. 316.
38. Ibid.
39. Simplicius. 1992. *On Aristotle's Physics, 4.105, 10-14*, trans. J. O. Urmason (Ithaca, NY: Cornell University Press).
40. Freeman, C. 2002. *The Closing of the Western Mind*, p. 317.
41. As noted above Aristotle postulated four causes of things: formal, material, efficient and final. This last is the purpose for which a thing is created. Modern evolutionists would deny a final cause for anything. See Galen, 1968, p. 9.
42. Marty, M. 2004. *Martin Luther* (New York: Penguin Group), p. 1.
43. Casper, M. 1993. Kepler, p. 22.
44. Kusukawa, S. 1995. *The Transformation of Natural Philosophy: The Case of Philip Melanchthon* (Cambridge: Cambridge University Press), p. 172.
45. Ibid.
46. This was later restated during Galileo's time: the business of the Church is to show men how to go to heaven rather than to show how the heavens go.
47. Durant, W. 1955. *The Reformation: A History of European Civilization from Wyclif to Calvin: 1300-1564* (New York: Simon & Schuster), p. 349.
48. Ibid., p. 352.
49. Ibid., p. 354.
50. Manuel, F. E. 1974. *The Religion of Isaac Newton: The Fremantle Lectures, 1973* (Oxford: Oxford University Press).
51. Fernandez-Armesto, P. 1997. *Truth: A Guide for the Perplexed* (New York: St. Martin's Press), pp. 70-74.
52. Garber, D. 1992. *Descartes' Metaphysical Physics* (Chicago: University of Chicago Press), p. 71.
53. De Bono, E. 1990. *I Am Right—You Are Wrong* (New York: Penguin), p. 198.
54. Veyene, P. 1988. *Did the Greeks Believe in Their Myths?* Trans. P. Wissing (Chicago: University of Chicago Press).
55. Lamont, C. 1957. *The Philosophy of Humanism* (New York: Philosophical Library), pp. 8-16.
56. Ibid., pp. 110-112.
57. Terracciano, A., et al. 2005. "National Character Does Not Reflect Mean Personality Trait Levels in 49 Cultures." *Science*, 310:96-100.

58. Bacon, F. 1960. *The New Organon* (Indianapolis, IN: Bobbs-Merrill), pp. 48-49.
59. Russell, B. 2005. "Why I Am Not a Christian," in *The Truth about the World*, ed. J. Rachels (New York: McGraw-Hill).
60. Dunn, J. 2004. *Elizabeth and Mary: Cousins, Rivals, Queens* (New York: Random House).
61. Cochrane, L. 1994. *Abelard of Bath: The First English Scientist* (London: British Museum Press), p. 17.
62. Armstrong, K. 2000. *The Battle for God*, p. xv-xviii.
63. De Bono, E. 1990. *I Am Right—You Are Wrong*, pp. 199-203.
64. Garber, J.J. 2005. "Jànos Bolyai, Non-Euclidean Geometry and the Concept of Space," CCWU Paper.
65. Jacker, C. 1966. *Window on the Unknown: A History of the Microscope* (New York: Charles Scribner's Sons) p. 35.
66. Apoptosis is the disintegration of cells into membrane-bound particles that are then eliminated by phagocytosis (gobbled up by white blood cells) or by shedding. Cells can replicate only so many times before they lose this ability. In other words, cells grow old.

Conclusion

Medicine, both ancient and medieval, found its roots in the only philosophical structure available to physicians of past ages. The intellectuals of these times were polymaths. They immersed themselves in all sciences then known. Both astronomy and medicine had their beginnings in prehistory. The oldest written records we know of come from Sumer (present day Iraq) where written language was first developed.[1] Undoubtedly, primitive astronomy and medicine antedate the written word, but Sumerian clay tablets give the first definite evidence of these two disciplines. Medical therapy began as a branch of botany. Herbal, along with animal and chemical therapies, were the mainstay of healing. Oftentimes, these were blended with magic and religion but the first glimmer of anything approaching medicine, as we think of it today, was discovered in a Sumerian herbal handbook.[2]

The first astronomical theories were Sumerian "philosophical cosmologies" dealing with the beginnings of the Universe. These were speculative constructs laden with gods and their creative powers, just as later Greek mythology portrayed them.[3] Out of this flowed the four humors—the essential sources of health and disease. It was their proper balance in the body, along with harmony of the heavens that provided the rational structure of medicine.

The transition from medieval to modern medicine provides one of the most fascinating stories of history, offering a penetrating glimpse into the workings of the human mind. It is, in essence, a study in the psychology of change. From a modern perspective, the persistence of ancient authority as the almost sole basis for "truth" is nearly incomprehensible. How could such obvious errors hold sway for so many centuries? One must recognize that past ages were times of great fear and insecurity. Little true knowledge of the workings of the world was available to the people of the past. After the fall of the Roman Empire, the day-to-day life of both peasant and noble was filled with unknowns. Disasters of all sorts, from pestilence to famine to war, were ever-present threats. Life was fragile and many died young; others suffered from chronic, debilitating mental and/or physical diseases. Insanity was a mysterious, awful affliction both baffling and untreatable. Someone had to be blamed for all these tragedies—the devil, some Manichean evil force, the immorality of people, a comet, a swampy miasma, the weather, bad water or the planets. The insecurity of the age made for multiple explanations for all the evils endured by humans. Sometimes the Church or even God was blamed and, indeed, cursed. All these maladies cried out for explanations but none was forthcoming except for the time-honored medical myths set forth by Hippocrates, Aristotle, and Galen centuries before. For the medieval mind there was an unshakeable mystique surrounding the ancient past. From serf to saint, bishop to pope and noble to academic, it was ancient authority that could not fail them. When the Black Death devastated Europe in the mid-fourteenth century, all the noted doctors of the day could only echo the astrology of Manilius and Ptolemy in blaming the plague on planetary conjunctions. Planets close together in the sky had increased power to affect the workings of the world and its inhabitants.

The "scientists" of the age had no technology or true science to help them find answers to these questions. The observational methods proposed by Hippocrates, Aristotle and Galen were doomed to failure because these men could not break loose from the speculative reasoning that seemed so "logical" to them. This is where emotions play such a major role in the flawed thinking of ancient authorities. All of us, at one time or another, are utterly convinced of the infallibility of our beliefs regarding one issue or another, this, in spite of data to the contrary. "Don't confuse me with the facts!" These "infallible" beliefs very often support some emotional, economic or social need we have. Virtually nothing will shake us from a rock-solid belief in these perceived "truths." We see this with many "hot-button" issues today—stem cell research, gay issues, abortion, Iraq, creationism, biblical interpretation and many more. Most of Germany fell victim to the rhetoric of Adolf Hitler for reasons of national pride. Whatever the genesis of these strongly held fictions, the fact remains that every age has had its myths to which it clings like a bulldog. To change is hard because it means letting go of some of our security and self-identity. In the end, scientists are only human. They are driven by the same desires that motivate us all. Only the exceptional few can topple a paradigm to begin a new age. A hundred years from now writers will be saying these same things about us and our beliefs. Today's paradigms will be incomprehensible to them and they will wonder how society could have held on so long to such antiquated views that today seem so "infallible."

Notes

1. Kramer, S. N. 1959. *History Begins at Sumer* (Garden City, NY: Doubleday), chapters 10 and 13.
2. Ibid. pp. 60-64.
3. Ibid., pp. 76-103.

Epilogue

During the twentieth and now twenty-first century, life has changed dramatically. The technological advances we have seen are mind-boggling, never to have been fully anticipated by even the most futuristic of futurists. This is true in the field of medicine as well. Even when I began studying medicine, we were only beginning to probe the depths of human health. The residuals of medieval medicine were still with us and in some ways are still around today in the alternate medicine practiced by many. This is not to ignore the fact that some herbal medicines are of benefit, though not to the extent espoused by some. But this is another whole topic too complex to review here.

The relationship between medicine and astronomy, however, persists but under an entirely new rubric. We have already encountered Fred Hoyle's *Diseases from Space,* which remains highly speculative at this juncture and is unlikely to see the light of a new scientific day. Space medicine, however, is alive and well and expanding in an exponential fashion. We are not only learning about the effect of weightlessness on humans and other animals but also delving into the very fundamentals of life itself. Our search for extraterrestrial life continues along with much speculation about what life is, where it can be found and what other forms of life there may be. Is all life water and carbon based? Or might there be multiple molecules with the potential to support biological systems very foreign to ours? Are there bacteria below the slushy surface of Europa or thermophiles living in the sulfurous volcanoes of Io? Did ancient life forms arrive from Mars eons ago to be found in Antarctica today? And if any of these questions are ultimately answered, what will this mean for the health of us humans? All these and many other questions remain. Only time will tell what the heavens hold in store for future medicine.

Appendix

Geocentrism is the belief that the Earth is at the center of the Universe; Deferents are the perfectly circular orbits the Sun, Moon, planets and stars move in around the Earth in the Ptolemaic construct. Epicycles are smaller circles that celestial objects follow as they move along the deferent. An equant is the central point of each deferent (orbit), which is not centered on the Earth but offset from it. The epicycle and equant are necessary adjustments in Ptolemy's system in order to allow for perfectly circular orbits, which, according to Aristotle, were the most "divine" and perfect geometric figures. Elliptical orbits would violate this rational and sacred structure of the Universe.

A.1

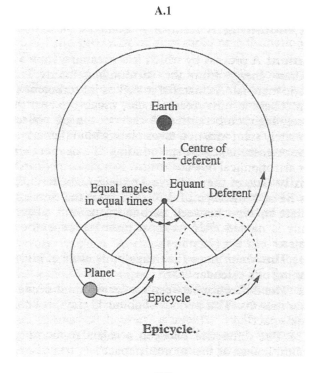

Epicycle.

The large circle is Ptolemy's deferent, representing the orbit of a planet, Sun or Moon. The epicycles are superimposed on the deferent. Each planet, the Sun and Moon, moves around the epicycle while the epicycle moves around the deferent. The whole system moves around the Earth. The Earth, however, is not at the center of the deferent. The center (focus) of the deferent is the equant. The equant and epicycles were needed by Ptolemy to account for the observed positions of the planets, Sun and Moon. Because the actual orbits of the planets, Sun and Moon are ellipses and not perfect circles, the focus of the deferent had to be offset from the Earth, so that the Earth was no longer the focus (center) of the deferent. The epicycles helped to account for the retrograde motion of the planets. This motion was actually due to the Earth passing the superior planets (outside Earth's orbit, i.e., Mars, Jupiter, and Saturn) as it (Earth) moved around the Sun. Because Ptolemy's system was geocentric, he could not explain these various motions of the planets without the epicycles and equants. Even with these adjustments, Kepler found significant variances from observed positions in both the Ptolemaic and Copernican systems and finally resolved the problem by postulating elliptical orbits for the Moon and planets within a heliocentric system.

References

Allen, R. H. 1963. *Star Names: Their Lore and Meaning* (New York: Dover).

Arano, L. C. 1996. *The Medieval Medical Handbook: Tacuinum Sanitatis*, trans. O. Ratti and A. Westbrook (New York: George Braziller).

Aratus. 1983. *Phaenomena* (Berkeley, CA: North Atlantic Books).

Aristotle. 1939. *On the Heavens*, Loeb Classics, trans. W. K. C. Guthrie (London: Harvard University Press).

Aristotle. 1942. *Generation of Animals*, Loeb Classics, trans. A. L. Peck (London: Harvard University Press).

Aristotle. 1952. *Aristotle's Metaphysics*, trans. R. Hope (New York: Columbia University Press).

Aristotle. 1960. *Metaphysics* (Ann Arbor: University of Michigan. Press).

Aristotle. 1984. *Meteorology, The Complete Works of Aristotle* (Princeton, NJ: Princeton University Press).

Aristotle. 1984. *De Anima, The Complete Works of Aristotle* (Princeton, NJ: Princeton University Press).

Aristotle. 1984. *On Generation and Corruption, The Complete Works of Aristotle* (Princeton, NJ: Princeton University Press).

Aristotle. 1984. *Prior Analytics, The Complete Works of Aristotle* (Princeton, NJ: Princeton University Press).

Aristotle. 1999. *Physics* (New York: Oxford University Press).

Armstrong, K. 1993. *A History of God: The 4000 Year Quest of Judaism, Christianity and Islam* (New York: Ballantine Books).

Armstrong, K. 1996. *Jerusalem: One City, Three Faiths* (New York: HarperCollins).

Armstrong, K. 2000. *The Battle for God* (New York: Ballantine Books).

Augustine, St. 1950. *City of God* (New York: Random House Modern Library).

Avicenna. 1930. *The Canon of Medicine*, trans. C. Gruner (London: Luzac and Co.).

Bacon, F. 1960. *The New Organon* (Indianapolis, IN: Bobbs-Merrill).

Bacon, R. 1998. *Opus majus*, trans. R. Belle (New York: Kesinger).

Bauval, R. and Gilbert, A. 1994. *The Orion Mystery* (New York: Three Rivers Press).

Best, M. R., and Brightman, F.H. 1999. *The Book of Secrets of Albertus Magnus* (York Beach, ME: Samuel Weiser).

Billings, A. 2000. *Corpus Hermeticum*, http://www.hermetic.com/texts/index.html.

Bingen, H. 1998. *Physica*, trans. P. Throop (Rochester, VT: Healing Arts Press).

Bramly, S. 1994. *Leonardo: The Artist and the Man*, trans. S. Reynolds (London: Penguin).

Burnet, T. 1685. *Hippocrates Contractus*, 1st Edition (Edinburgh, Scotland: J. Reid).

Burnet, T. 1743. *Hippocrates Contractus*, 2nd Edition (London, Car. Davis and John Whiston, Fleetstreet).

Cahane, H. and Cavender, N. 1998. *Logic and Contemporary Rhetoric: The Use of Reason in Everyday Life* (New York: Wadsworth).

Capella, M. 1977, Martianus Capella and the Seven Liberal Arts, trans. W. H. Stahl and B. L. Burge (New York: Columbia University Press).

Casper, M. 1993. *Kepler*, trans. and ed. C. D. Hellman (New York: Dover).

Castleden, R. 1987. *The Stonehenge People* (New York: Routledge and Kegan Paul).

Celsus. 1989. *De Medicina*, trans. W.G. Spencer, Loeb Classics (Cambridge, MA: Harvard University Press).

Challener, S. 2000. 195th AAS meeting, #92.01.

Chaucer, G. 1977. *The Canterbury Tales*, trans. N. Coghill (New York: Penguin).

Christianson, J. R. 2000. *On Tycho's Island: Tycho Brahe and his Assistants, 1590-1601* (New York: Cambridge University Press).

Cicero, M. T. 1997. *On Divination*, trans. C. D. Yonge (Amherst, NY: Prometheus Books).

Clegg, B. 2003. *The First Scientist: A Life of Roger Bacon* (New York: Carroll and Graf).

Cochrane, L. 1994. *Abelard of Bath: The First English Scientist* (London: British Museum Press).

Cooke, I. 1987. *Mermaid to Merrymaid: Journey to the Stones* (Over Wallop, UK: BAS Printers).

Copernicus, N. 1995. *On the Revolutions of Heavenly Spheres* (Amherst, NY: Prometheus).

Coulston, C. 1997. *Pierre-Simon LaPlace 1749-1827: A Life in Exact Science* (Princeton, NJ: Princeton University Press).

Cramer, F. H. 1954. *Astrology in Roman Law and Politics* (Philadelphia, PA: American Philosophical Society).

Crombie, A. C. 1995. *The History of Science from Augustine to Galileo* (New York: Dover).

Crowe, M. J. 1990. *Theories of the World from Antiquity to the Copernican Revolution* (New York: Dover).

Crellin, J. K. and Philpott, J. 1989. *A Reference Guide to Medicinal Plants: Herbal Medicine Past and Present* (Durham, NC: Duke University Press).

Da Vinci, L. 1983. *Leonardo on the Human Body*, trans. and text, O'Malley, C.D. and Saunders, J.B. de C.M. (New York: Dover).

Da Vinci, L. 2005. *Leonardo's Notebooks*, ed. H. Anna Suh (New York: Black Dog and Leventhal).

De Bono, E. 1990. *I Am Right—You Are Wrong* (New York: Penguin).

Debus, A. G. 1970. "Harvey and Fludd: The Irrational Factor in the Rational Science of the Seventeenth Century," *Journal of the History of Biology*, 3, 81.

Dick, H. C. 1946. "Students of Physic and Astrology: A Survey of Astrological Medicine in the Age of Science," *Journal of the History of Medicine and Allied Sciences*, 1, 300.

Dunn, J. 2004. *Elizabeth and Mary: Cousins, Rivals, Queens* (New York: Random House).

Duggan, C. 1994. *A Concise History of Italy* (Cambridge: Cambridge University Press).

Durant, W. 1955. *The Renaissance: A History of Civilization in Italy from 1304-1576 A.D.* (New York: Simon and Schuster).

Durant, W. 1957. *The Reformation: A History of European Civilization from Wyclif to Calvin: 1300-1564* (New York: Simon and Schuster).

Edelstein, E. and Edelstein, L. 1998. *Asclepius: Collection and Interpretation of the Testimonies* (Baltimore, MD: Johns Hopkins University Press).

Edelstein, L. 1943. "Andreas Vesalius: The Humanist," Bull. *History of Medicine*, 14:547-61.

Edelstein, L. 1967. *Ancient Medicine*, ed. O. Temkin and C. L. Temkin (Baltimore, MD: Johns Hopkins University Press).

Eddy, J. A. 1978, *In Search of Ancient Astronomy*, ed. E. C. Krupp (New York: McGraw-Hill).

Edwards, I. E. S. 1903. *The Pyramids of Egypt* (London/New York: Penguin).

Ellis, P. B. 1994. *The Druids* (New York: William B. Eerdmans).

Engle, E., and Lott, A. S. 1979. *Man in Flight* (Annapolis, MD: Leeward). Fernandez-Armesto, P. 1997. *Truth: A Guide for the Perplexed* (New York: St. Martin's Press).

Fernandez, Y. R. et al. 2002. "Thermal Properties of Centaurs Asbolus and Chiron," *Astronomical Journal*, 123, 1050

Firmicus, M. 1973. *Mathesos: Ancient Astrology: Theory and Practice*, trans. J. R. Bram (Park Ridge, NJ: Noyes Press).

Fludd, R. 2001. *Robert Fludd*, ed. W. Huffman (Berkeley, CA: North Atlantic Books).

Freeman, C. 2002. *The Closing of the Western Mind: The Rise of Faith and the Fall of Reason* (New York: Vintage Books).

Galen, C. 1929. *On the Natural Faculties*, trans. A. J. Brock (Cambridge, MA: Harvard University Press).

Galen, C. 1968. *On the Usefulness of the Parts of the Body*, trans. M. Tallmadge May (Ithaca, NY: Cornell, University Press).

Galen, C. 1979. *On Prognosis*, trans. V. Nutton (Berlin, Germany: Akademie-Verlag).

Galen, C. 1997. *Galen: Selected Works*, trans. P.N. Singer (Oxford, UK: Oxford University Press).

Galilei, G. 1957. *Discoveries and Opinions of Galileo*, trans. S. Drake (Garden City, NY: Doubleday Anchor Books).

Galilei, G. 1957. "Starry Messenger," trans. S. Drake in *Discoveries and Opinions of Galileo* (Garden City, NY: Doubleday-Anchor).

Galilei, G. 2001. *Dialogue Concerning the Two Chief World Systems* (New York: Modern Library).

Garber, D. 1992. *Descartes' Metaphysical Physics* (Chicago: University of Chicago Press).

Garber, J. J. 2002, "Cepheid Variables: A Philosophical and Scientific Odyssey," University of Western Sydney, History of Astronomy Paper.

Garber, J. J. 2005. "Jànos Bolyai, Non-Euclidean Geometry and the Concept of Space," CCWU Paper.

Gottfried, R. S. 1983. *The Black Death* (New York: Macmillan Free Press).

Grant, E. 1996. *Planets, Stars, and Orbs: The Medieval Cosmos, 1200-1687* (New York: Cambridge University Press).

Guthrie, K. S. 1987. *The Pythagorean Source Book and Library* (Grand Rapids, MI: Phanes Press).

Haggard, H. W. 1962. *The Doctor in History* (Freeport, NY: Books for Libraries Press).

Harvey, W. 1993. *On the Motion of the Heart and Blood in Animals*, trans. R. Willis (Amherst, NY: Prometheus Books).

Heath, T. L. 1991. *Greek Astronomy* (New York: Dover).

Heraclitus. 2003. *Fragments*, trans. B. Haxton (New York: Penguin).

Hesiod. 1983. *Theogony and Works and Days*, trans. M. L. West (Oxford, UK: Oxford University Press).

Hibbert, C. 1995. *Rome: The Biography of a City* (New York: Penguin).

Hippocrates. 1923. *Writings*, vols. I-IV, Loeb Classics, trans. W. H. S. Jones (London/New York: Harvard University Press).

Hippocrates. 1978. *Hippocratic Writings*, trans. J. Chadwick and W. N. Mann, ed. G. E. R. Lloyd (New York: Penguin Books).

Hossein, S. 1978. *An Introduction to Islamic Cosmological Doctrine* (Boulder, CO: Shambhala Press).

Hoyle, F. 1979. *Diseases from Space* (New York: Harper and Row).

Jacker, C. 1966. *Window on the Unknown: A History of the Microscope* (New York: Charles Scribner's Sons).

Johnson, P. 1999. *The Civilization of Ancient Egypt* (New York: HarperCollins).

Jones, P.M. 1998. *Medieval Medicine in Illuminated Manuscripts* (London: British Library).

Kepler, J. 1995. *Epitome of Copernican Astronomy and Harmonies of the World* (Amherst, NY: Prometheus Books).

Koerner, D., and Levay, S. 2000. *Here Be Dragons: The Scientific Quest for Extraterrestrial Life* (New York: Oxford University Press).

Kramer, S. N. 1959. *History Begins at Sumer* (Garden City, NY: Doubleday).

Koval, C. T. 1979. "The Discovery and Orbit of (2060) Chiron, IAUS," *Dynamics of the Solar System*, 81, 245.

Kuhn, T. S. 1977. *The Essential Tension* (Chicago, IL: Chicago University Press).

Kusukawa, S. 1995. *The Transformation of Natural Philosophy: The Case of Philip Melanchthon* (Cambridge, UK: Cambridge University Press).

Lamont, C. 1957. *The Philosophy of Humanism* (New York: Philosophical Library).

Lambridis, H. 1976. *Empedocles* (University, AL: University of Alabama Press).

Lindberg, D. C. 1976. *Theories of Vision* (Chicago, IL: University of Chicago Press).

Lindberg, D. C. 1978. *Science in the Middle Ages* (Chicago, IL: University of Chicago Press).

Lindbloom, G. A. 1978, *Descartes and Medicine* (Amsterdam, Neth.: Rodopi).

Longrigg, J. 1993. *Greek Rational Medicine: Philosophy and Medicine from Alcmaeon to the Alexandrians* (New York: Routledge).

Lucretius. 1986. *On the Nature of the Universe*, trans. R. E. Latham (New York: Penguin Books).

Maimonides, M. 1956. *The Guide for the Perplexed*, trans. M. Friedlander (New York: Dover)

Manilius. 1927. *Astronomica*, Loeb Classics, trans. G. P. Goold (London/New York: Harvard University Press).

Manuel, F. E. 1974. *The Religion of Isaac Newton: The Fremantle Lectures*, 1973 (Oxford, UK: Oxford University Press).

Marks, G. and Beatty, W. K. 1976. *Epidemics* (New York: Charles Scribner's Sons).

Marty, M. 2004. *Martin Luther* (New York: Penguin Group).

Mayerson, P. 1971. *Classical Mythology in Literature, Art and Music* (New York: John Wiley and Sons).

McCluskey, S. C. 1998 *Astronomers and Cultures in Early Medieval Europe* (New York, NY: Cambridge University Press).

McEvoy, J. 2000. *Robert Grosseteste* (New York: Oxford University Press).

Moscati, S. 2001. *The Phoenicians* (New York: Gardner Books).

Nazr, S. H. 1978. *An Introduction to Islamic Cosmological Doctrines* (Boulder, CO: Shambhala).

Neugebauer, O. and van Hoesen, H. B. 1959. *Greek Horoscopes* (Philadelphia, PA: American Philosophical Society).

Neugebauer, O. 1969. *The Exact Sciences in Antiquity* (New York: Dover).

Newton, I. 1934. *Principia*: Vol. I, *The Motion of Bodies* (Berkeley, CA: University of California Press).

Nicholl, C. 2004. *Leonardo da Vinci: Flights of the Mind* (London: Viking Penguin).

Nuland, S.W. 1989, *Doctors: The Biography of Medicine* (New York: Vintage Books).

O'Boyle, C. 1998. *The Art of Medicine: Medical Teaching at the University of Paris, 1250-1400* (Boston, MA: Brill).

O'Neill, Y. V. 1969, Chaucer and medicine, JAMA, 208: 78-82.

Orion, R. 1999. *Astrology for Dummies* (New York: IDG Books Worldwide).

Pagels, E. 1979. *The Gnostic Gospels* (New York: Vintage Books).

Paracelsus. 1983. *Hermetic Astronomy* (Edmonds, WA: Sure Fire Press).

Paracelsus. 1999. *Essential Readings*, trans. N. Goodrick-Clarke (Berkeley, CA: North Atlantic Books)

Pedersen, O. 1985. *In Quest of Sacrobosco, Journal of the History of Astronomy*, 16, 175.

Plato. 1977. *Timaeus and Critias* (London: Penguin Books).

Plato. 1978. *The Republic of Plato*, trans. F.M. Cornford (New York: Oxford University Press).

Pliny. 1991. *Natural History: A Selection*, trans. J. Healy (New York: Penguin).

Pope, H. 1961. *Augustine of Hippo* (Garden City, NY: Image Books).

Porter, R. 1997. *The Greatest Benefit to Mankind: A Medical History of Humanity* (New York: W.W. Norton and Co.).

Ptolemy, C. 1976. *Tetrabiblos* (North Hollywood, CA: Symbols and Signs).

Ptolemy, C. 1998. *Almagest* (Princeton, NJ: Princeton University Press).

Rawcliffe, C. 1999. *Medicine and Society in Later Medieval England* (London: Sandpiper).

Rosen, R. 1994. *Copernicus and the Scientific Revolution* (Malabar, FL: R. E. Krieger).

Russell, B. 2005. "Why I Am Not a Christian," in *The Truth about the World*, ed. J. Rachels (New York: McGraw-Hill).

Ruggles, C. and Hoskin, M. 1999. *The Cambridge Concise History of Astronomy*, ed. M. Hoskin (Cambridge: Cambridge University Press).

Sambursky, S. 1956. *The Physical World of the Greeks*, trans. M. Dagut (Princeton, NJ: Princeton University Press).

Seneca. 1969. *Letters from a Stoic* (New York: Penguin).

Simplicius. 1992. *Simplicius: On Aristotle's Physics 4.1-5*, 10-14.

Siraisi, N. G. 1990. *Medieval and Renaissance Medicine* (Chicago: University of Chicago).

Stigler, S. M. 1986. *The History of Statistics: The Measurement of Uncertainty before 1900* (Cambridge, MA: Belknap Press of Harvard University Press).

Stigler, S. M. 1999. *Statistics on the Table: The History of Statistical Concepts and Methods* (Cambridge, MA: Harvard University Press).

Strathern, P. 2000. *Mendeleyev's Dream: The Quest for the Elements* (New York: St. Martin's Press).

Temkin, O, 1973. *Galenism: Rise and Decline of a Medical Philosophy* (Ithaca, NY: Cornell University Press).

Terracciano, A. et al. 2005. "National Character Does Not Reflect Mean Personality Trait Levels in 49 Cultures," *Science*, 310: 96-100.

Tester, S. J. 1999. *A History of Western Astrology* (Rochester, NY: Bondell Press).

Thatcher, O. J. 1901. *The Library of Original Sources* (Milwaukee, WI: University Research Extension). Internet Medieval Source Book.

Thompson, K. H., and Orvig, C. 2003. "The Boon and Bane of Metal Ions in Medicine," *Science*, 300: 936-939.

Wilson, C. 1980. *The Starseekers* (Garden City, NY: Doubleday and Co.).

Witzel, T. 2003. *Catholic Encyclopedia* XIII (New York: Online Edition).

Woolley, B. 2004. *Heal Thyself: Nicholas Culpeper and the Seventeenth-Century Struggle to Bring Medicine to the People* (New York: HarperCollins).

Wright, M. R. 1995. *Empedocles: The Extant Fragments* (Indianapolis, IN: Hackett).

Index